Pharmacy
Calculations
for Technicians

Fifth Edition

Instructor's Guide

Don A. Ballington • Tova Wiegand-Green

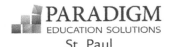
PARADIGM
EDUCATION SOLUTIONS
St. Paul

Managing Editor	Brenda M. Palo
Developmental Editor	Nancy Papsin
Production Editor	Katherine Lee
Cover Designer	Jaana Bykonich
Text Designer	Jaana Bykonich
Illustrator	S4Carlisle (pages 69–183)
Cover Images	iStockphoto/BahadirTanriover (top left), George Brainard (top right), Shutterstock/ Ragne Kabanova (bottom left)

Care has been taken to verify the accuracy of information presented in this book. However, the authors, editors, and publisher cannot accept responsibility for Web, e-mail, newsgroup, or chat room subject matter or content, or for consequences from application of the information in this book, and make no warranty, expressed or implied, with respect to its content.

Trademarks: Some of the product names and company names included in this book have been used for identification purposes only and may be trademarks or registered trade names of their respective manufacturers and sellers. The authors, editors, and publisher disclaim any affiliation, association, or connection with, or sponsorship or endorsement by, such owners.

We have made every effort to trace the ownership of all copyrighted material and to secure permission from copyright holders. In the event of any question arising as to the use of any material, we will be pleased to make the necessary corrections in future printings. Thanks are due to the aforementioned authors, publishers, and agents for permission to use the materials indicated.

ISBN 978-0-76385-219-1 (IG)
ISBN 978-0-76385-222-1 (IG & CD)

© Paradigm Publishing, Inc.
875 Montreal Way
St. Paul, MN 55102
E-mail: educate@emcp.com
Web site: www.emcp.com

Printed in the United States of America

22 21 20 19 18 17 16   4 5 6 7 8 9 10

Contents

Chapter Practice Test Answer Keys 191

Additional Assessments. 201

Answer Keys for Additional Assessments. 232

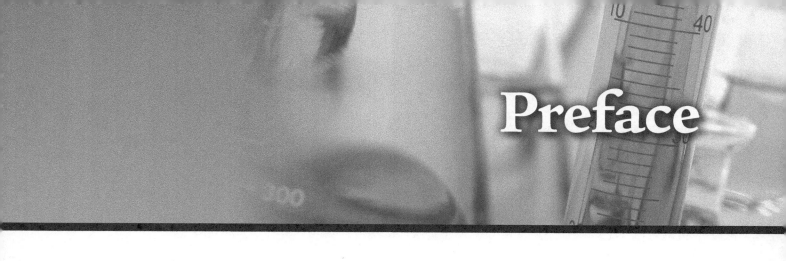

Preface

This supplement has been prepared for instructors who are using *Pharmacy Calculations for Technicians, Fifth Edition*, by Don A. Ballington and Tova Wiegand-Green. This resource will help plan a comprehensive course that provides aspiring pharmacy technicians with the essential knowledge and skills needed for a successful career as pharmacy paraprofessionals.

The *Instructor's Guide* includes sections on Planning the Course, Pharmacy Calculations Pretest, Chapter Lessons, Handouts, Chapter Review Answer Keys, Chapter Practice Test Answer Keys, and Additional Assessments:

- The Planning the Course section offers a framework for instructors to follow to help them establish course outcomes, determine course content and structure (including suggested syllabus models), and develop instructional approaches and assessment strategies.
- The Pharmacy Calculations Pretest provides instructors with a baseline assessment of students' math skills in such areas as fractions, decimals, ratios, and percentages.
- The Chapter Lessons section provides learning objectives based on the *ASHP Model Curriculum for Pharmacy Technician Training, Second Edition*. This section also offers chapter overviews, plan-ahead tips, instructional approaches, and suggested activities to supplement student textbook instruction.
- The Handouts section provides a series of worksheets that contain measuring devices commonly used in pharmacy practice. These handouts correspond to specific problems in the student textbook. Students are asked to solve the problems and then use the answers to determine the volumes that should be filled in on the measuring devices. The handout answer keys are also provided for instructors in this section.
- The Chapter Review Answer Keys section supplies the correct answers for the end-of-chapter exercises: Assessing Comprehension, Finding Solutions, and Sampling the Certification Exam.
- The Chapter Practice Test Answer Keys offer the correct answers for the Chapter Practice Tests that appear in the student textbook.
- The Additional Assessments section provides instructors with two versions of chapter tests (Version A and Version B) that assess students' understanding of content. Providing two versions gives instructors the flexibility of using one or both tests with their students. The answer keys for both versions are also provided in this section.

All of the resources from the print *Instructor's Guide* are available in electronic form on the accompanying Instructor Resources CD and on the password-protected instructor's section of the Internet Resource Center at www.paradigmcollege.net/pharmcalc5e. Instructors can download materials for use in their courses.

The authors and editorial staff encourage feedback on the text and its supplements. Please reach us by clicking the "Contact Us" button at www.emcp.com.

Planning the Course

Most educators would agree that the key to teaching a successful course is careful, thorough planning. And, as noted in *Exceptional Teaching: Ideas in Action*, published by Paradigm Publishing, "Instructors assess, plan, implement, and evaluate... repeatedly. They do this based on many of the factors that make teaching learner-centered and on several other variables. Before students even think about entering or logging into the classroom, instructors make decisions about the course. These begin with identifying the heart of the course. That is, what, exactly, are the most important outcomes that students should achieve? And what plan of action can the instructor devise that will help ensure those outcomes?" Thinking through a course action plan typically includes four phases:

1. Developing the course outcomes
2. Determining the course delivery mode and structure (dividing the course into parts, each with outcomes)
3. Selecting the course's instructional approach, resources, and activities
4. Developing an assessment strategy

Developing Course Outcomes

In developing course outcomes for any course, consider the following key issues:

- While delivering the course, keep in mind how the learner will
  - most effectively receive feedback
  - discover whether his or her work is satisfactory
  - be best served by instruction that suits her or his dominant learning styles
- When this course is over, consider how the learner could be permanently changed for the better because your instruction developed his or her
  - knowledge (in which broad or specific categories?)
  - independent learning skills
  - communication skills (for facility within which discourse communities?)
  - higher-order thinking
  - decision-making skills (based on what type of scenarios or data?)
  - technical literacy
- As a learner enters the professional realm, how should this course have prepared him or her to succeed given the
  - scope of conditions under which the work is performed
  - decision-making challenges on the job
  - varied communication skills required
  - ongoing demands to update his or her knowledge and technical skills

Considering the preceding questions, a set of end-of-course outcomes for a one-semester *Pharmacy Calculations for Technicians* course could include the following items, stated as performances:

- Understand subdivisions of numbers, number systems, estimating, and accuracy.
- Demonstrate the relationship between units of measurement, and use their correct abbreviations.
- Describe the use of ratios, percents, and proportions in pharmacy practice.
- Understand the ratio-proportion and dimensional analysis methods in performing pharmacy calculations.
- Calculate doses related to the administration of medication utilizing various systems of measurement.
- Accurately read drug labels for amount of active ingredient contained in a measured amount of medication, and calculate the amount of medication to dispense for a specific dose.
- Calculate the quantity of active ingredient in a percentage solution and solid mixture.
- Calculate the amount of concentrate and diluent needed for a stock dilution compound.
- Calculate age- and weight-specific drug doses or dose range when given recommended dose information.
- Use a nomogram to estimate a patient's body surface area (BSA), and use that BSA to calculate a patient-specific dose of medication.
- Understand the types of intravenous (IV) sets, and calculate IV drip rates and flow rates.
- Calculate the amount of ingredients needed to enlarge or reduce a formula.
- Use the alligation method to calculate the amount of two strengths of active ingredient needed to prepare a product whose concentration lies between the two extremes.
- Determine the amount of two ingredients using the weight-in-weight (w/w) formula.
- Calculate the least weighable quantity when given the specifications of the measuring device being used.
- Understand how to prepare a special dilution.
- Calculate business application needs such as percent markup, percent profit, overhead, profit, gross profit, percentage of average wholesale price (AWP), capitation, days' supply of inventory, and inventory maintenance ordering with minimums and maximums.

Determining the Course Delivery Mode and Structure

Whether you are planning a traditional on-campus course or a hybrid course that incorporates online (distance-learning) course work with lab instruction, the core considerations are the same. Chief among them are the course outcomes, class schedule, student characteristics, course subject matter, and available resources. The different instructional approaches between the delivery modes, however, create distinct needs you must address in the planning stage. Because hybrid courses represent a minority of college classes—although a growing minority—they offer special challenges for instructors, particularly educators new to this delivery mode.

Hybrid Course: Special Considerations

A critical challenge in teaching a hybrid course is the issue of interacting with the students. How will you communicate with them? How will they submit assignments and tests? How will you deliver feedback? How will you get to know your students?

Here are some additional questions to consider when planning a hybrid course, as suggested in *Exceptional Teaching*:

1. What course management system will be used: Webcourses, Moodle, or some other platform?

2. What portion of the course will be offered online and what will be done in the lab? Will you teach a course where students work independently offline and use the course management system to review course outcomes, the syllabus, assignment due dates; communicate with the instructor; take online quizzes; transmit completed work; and participate in chat sessions?

3. Will you have an on-campus orientation meeting with your students at the beginning of the course? In some situations, because of the distance factor, students will not be able to come to campus. However, if feasible, by all means conduct an orientation meeting. Many students will likely have the same questions that can be answered at one time, and the face-to-face contact at an orientation will benefit both you and the students.

4. Will the students come to the campus or school to take exams? If not, will students be directed to off-site locations where exams can be administered to verify that the person taking the exam is indeed the person getting credit for the course? It is critical that this step be set up before the hybrid course begins.

5. What PC configuration and/or software requirements must a student have to participate in your hybrid course?

Course Structure

Once you have determined your course delivery mode, you must consider the overall structure of your course and the goals that you want your curriculum to meet. The text is designed for the student with little or no experience in pharmacy practice to prepare for successful completion of the Pharmacy Technician Certification Board (PTCB) exam or its equivalent. The book is aligned with the American Society of Health-Systems Pharmacists' (ASHP) Model Curriculum for Pharmacy Technician Training as well as the most recent guidelines published by the United States Pharmacopoeia (USP) as contained in Chapters <795> and <797>. The text, supplemented with laboratory and practical experiences in contemporary practice, will prepare the student for employment as a knowledgeable and trained paraprofessional in either community or institutional pharmacy. Instructors are encouraged to consider applying for national accreditation with ASHP if their program meets the published standards with a minimum of 600 hours of instruction over 15 weeks or more. See www.ashp.org for additional information.

Course Design Considerations

Textbook authors typically design their content to align with the most popular course structure for a particular subject, and they develop syllabus plans that correlate with that framework. In this situation, much of your basic planning is therefore completed, and you may only need to modify the course structure and the resulting syllabus slightly. If you are in a position to develop a plan or modify an existing structure, consider these questions:

- What topics are essential for demonstrating the course outcomes?
- Is this the only course that will address this subject and skill set?
- What do students already know about the subject, its subtopics, and its associated skill set? What can they learn on their own, independent of your direct instruction?
- Where in each topic will the instruction "begin" and "end"?

A comprehensive syllabus should help you and your students prepare for each part of the class. Syllabi are useful for both traditional, on-campus courses as well as courses that are delivered in a hybrid format. Generally, the following elements are included in a syllabus:

1. Course identifying data
2. Prerequisites
3. Instructor contact information
4. Course outcomes
5. Required course resources
6. Major assignments
7. Grade composition
8. Class structure
9. Course schedule
10. College/school requirements

Figure 1 is an example of a traditional, on-campus course syllabus designed for a one-semester, 16-week course that meets three times a week using *Pharmacy Calculations for Technicians, Fifth Edition*. Figure 2 shows a schedule for a quarter-based course comprised of two 10-week sessions. You can use these documents as a starting point for your own course syllabus. The assignments column is left blank for the instructor to fill in or for students to fill in. Having students fill in the assignments themselves encourages accountability and attention to detail. Pertinent information about the apothecary system has been included on handouts that are available for instructors on the Internet Resource Center.

Textbook Format

Pharmacy Calculations for Technicians, Fifth Edition uses a stepped approach to learning. The textbook begins with a review of basic mathematical concepts such as fractions, decimals, percents, ratios, and number systems. Each subsequent chapter builds in difficulty, with Chapter 8 addressing more complex pharmacy calculations such as preparing parenteral medications and special dilutions. Chapter 9 allows students to use their math skills for a different application: the business aspect of operating a pharmacy.

The chapters themselves are organized by sections that focus on a specific mathematical concept. At the end of each section is a problem set, providing students with plenty of practice in that particular skill set. In addition, end-of-chapter exercises and a chapter practice test further reinforce the math concepts presented in each chapter.

All in all, the textbook provides your students with the essential mathematics concepts and calculation skills that they will need to prepare drug doses in both community and institutional pharmacy settings.

Assessments and Certifications

Another consideration when preparing your course syllabus is determining the types of assessments you want to implement and the instructional goals they serve. For example, to prepare your students to pass the mid-semester and final exams, you may wish to create quizzes based on the material presented in the chapter. Quizzes can be formulated using the **EXAM**VIEW® Assessment Suite program (found on the Instructor Resources CD) and administered to students according to the timeline suggested in the course schedule. Assessments have also been created for instructor use in the Additional Assessments section of this print supplement. There, you will find additional chapter tests for you to use. Each chapter test provides two versions—Version A and Version B—so that you have the flexibility to administer either exam.

A final consideration when creating assessments for your course syllabus is preparing students for the PTCE and ExCPT certification exams. With that goal in mind, Paradigm Publishing has a separate textbook, *Certification Exam Review for Pharmacy Technicians, Third Edition*, that offers test-taking strategies and practice tests for students. This new edition has been substantially restructured to align with the nine knowledge domains identified by the PTCB in its blueprint for the exam.

Course Syllabus Models

The following syllabus models are tailored specifically to the achievement of course outcomes within a designated time frame.

One 16-Week Semester, Syllabus Example

Course Description

This course teaches students the essential pharmacy calculations that are performed in a pharmacy setting. The primary objective is to develop problem-solving skills, including how to use information from written prescriptions, hospital orders, and labels of products available in a pharmacy. Pharmacy calculations typically used on a daily basis in retail and institutional pharmacies are emphasized. Business terms and business math skills essential to pharmacy practice—as well as calculations to determine inventory and purchasing needs, profit margins, and inventory control—are also covered.

Course Outcomes

- Understand subdivisions of numbers, number systems, estimating, and accuracy.
- Demonstrate the relationship between units of measurement, and use their correct abbreviations.
- Describe the use of ratios, percents, and proportions in pharmacy practice.
- Understand the ratio-proportion and dimensional analysis methods in performing pharmacy calculations.
- Calculate doses related to the administration of medication utilizing various systems of measurement.
- Accurately read drug labels for amount of active ingredient contained in a measured amount of medication, and calculate the amount of medication to dispense for a specific dose.
- Calculate the quantity of active ingredient in a percentage solution and solid mixture.
- Calculate the amount of concentrate and diluent needed for a stock dilution compound.
- Calculate age- and weight-specific drug doses or dose range when given recommended dose information.
- Use a nomogram to estimate a patient's body surface area (BSA), and use that BSA to calculate a patient-specific dose of medication.
- Understand the types of intravenous (IV) sets, and calculate IV drip rates and flow rates.
- Calculate the amount of ingredients needed to enlarge or reduce a formula.
- Use the alligation method to calculate the amount of two strengths of active ingredient needed to prepare a product whose concentration lies between the two extremes.
- Determine the amount of two ingredients using the weight-in-weight (w/w) formula.
- Calculate the least weighable quantity when given the specifications of the measuring device being used.
- Understand how to prepare a special dilution.
- Calculate business application needs such as percent markup, percent profit, overhead, profit, gross profit, percentage of average wholesale price (AWP), capitation, days' supply of inventory, and inventory maintenance ordering with minimums and maximums.

Prerequisites

None

Instructor Contact Information

    Name:
    Office Phone:
    Office E-mail:
    Office Location:
    Office Hours:

Required Course Resources

Pharmacy Calculations for Technicians, Fifth Edition with Study Partner CD
www.paradigmcollege.net/pharmcalc5e

Study Time

Approximately six to eight hours per week of study or homework time outside of class is recommended for successful completion of course requirements.

Suggested Grading

Final grades will be calculated as follows:

Attendance	5%
Homework, including Study Partner quizzes (reported mode)	5%
Homework Assignments	20%
Weekly Quizzes	20%
Chapter Tests	20%
Comprehensive Final Exam	30%

College and Course Policy Information

- This college conforms to the provisions of the Americans with Disabilities Act. You are invited to report any special needs to your instructor.
- Your attendance and participation are expected at all class sessions. Excessive unexcused absences may affect your final grade or result in dismissal from the class.
- Cell phone use (ringing, answering, text messaging) is not allowed in class.
- We subscribe to the college policy on academic honesty found in the school catalog.

Course Schedule

Week	Topic	Assignments
1	Introduction and Pretest	
2	Chapter 1 Fractions, Number Systems, Decimals, Estimates, Significant Figures, Time	
3	Chapter 2 Ratios, Percent, Proportions, Percentage Error	
4	Chapter 3 Prescription Orders, Prescription Directions	
5	Chapter 4 Metric Units, Conversions	
6	Chapter 4 Problem Solving, Customized Doses	
7	Chapter 5 Household Measure, Oral Doses, Temperature	
8	Chapter 6 Parenteral Injections and Infusions	

Week	Topic	Assignments
9	Chapter 6 Other Units of Measure, Using Powdered Medication	
10	Chapter 7 Percentage and Ratio Strength Dilutions	
11	Chapter 7 IV Flow Rates, Drop Factor and Infusion Rates	
12	Chapter 8 Compounded Formulas, Alligations	
13	Chapter 8 Weight-in-Weight (w/w) Calculations, Special Dilutions	
14	Chapter 9 Business Math, Insurance Reimbursement	
15	Chapter 9 Inventory Review for Final	
16	Comprehensive Final Examination	

Two 10-Week Quarters, Syllabus Example

Course Description

This course teaches students the essential pharmacy calculations that are performed in a pharmacy setting. The primary objective is to develop problem-solving skills, including how to use information from written prescriptions, hospital orders, and labels of products available in a pharmacy. Pharmacy calculations typically used on a daily basis in retail and institutional pharmacies are emphasized. Business terms and business math skills essential to pharmacy practice—as well as calculations to determine inventory and purchasing needs, profit margins, and inventory control—are also covered.

Course Outcomes

- Understand subdivisions of numbers, number systems, estimating, and accuracy.
- Demonstrate the relationship between units of measurement, and use their correct abbreviations.
- Describe the use of ratios, percents, and proportions in pharmacy practice.
- Understand the ratio-proportion and dimensional analysis methods in performing pharmacy calculations.
- Calculate doses related to the administration of medication utilizing various systems of measurement.
- Accurately read drug labels for amount of active ingredient contained in a measured amount of medication, and calculate the amount of medication to dispense for a specific dose.

- Calculate the quantity of active ingredient in a percentage solution and solid mixture.
- Calculate the amount of concentrate and diluent needed for a stock dilution compound.
- Calculate age- and weight-specific drug doses or dose range when given recommended dose information.
- Use a nomogram to estimate a patient's body surface area (BSA), and use that BSA to calculate a patient-specific dose of medication.
- Understand the types of intravenous (IV) sets, and calculate IV drip rates and flow rates.
- Calculate the amount of ingredients needed to enlarge or reduce a formula.
- Use the alligation method to calculate the amount of two strengths of active ingredient needed to prepare a product whose concentration lies between the two extremes.
- Determine the amount of two ingredients using the weight-in-weight (w/w) formula.
- Calculate the least weighable quantity when given the specifications of the measuring device being used.
- Understand how to prepare a special dilution.
- Calculate business application needs such as percent markup, percent profit, overhead, profit, gross profit, percentage of average wholesale price (AWP), capitation, days' supply of inventory, and inventory maintenance ordering with minimums and maximums.

Prerequisites

None

Instructor Contact Information

Name:
Office Phone:
Office E-mail:
Office Location:
Office Hours:

Required Course Resources

Pharmacy Calculations for Technicians, Fifth Edition with Study Partner CD
www.paradigmcollege.net/pharmcalc5e

Study Time

Approximately six to eight hours per week of study or homework time outside of class is recommended for successful completion of course requirements.

Suggested Grading

Final grades will be calculated as follows:

Attendance	5%
Homework, including Study Partner quizzes (reported mode)	5%
Homework Assignments	20%
Weekly Quizzes	20%
Chapter Tests	20%
Comprehensive Final Exam	30%

College and Course Policy Information

- This college conforms to the provisions of the Americans with Disabilities Act. You are invited to report any special needs to your instructor.
- Your attendance and participation are expected at all class sessions. Excessive unexcused absences may affect your final grade or result in dismissal from the class.
- Cell phone use (ringing, answering, text messaging) is not allowed in class.
- We subscribe to the college policy on academic honesty found in the school catalog.

Course Schedule

First 10 Weeks

Week	Topic	Homework Assignment
1	Introduction and Pretest	
2	Chapter 1 Fractions, Number Systems, Decimals	
3	Chapter 1 Estimates, Significant Figures, Time	
4	Chapter 2 Ratios, Percent	
5	Chapter 2 Proportions, Percentage Error	
6	Chapter 3 Prescription Orders, Prescription Directions	
7	Chapter 4 Metric Units	
8	Chapter 4 Conversions, Problem Solving	
9	Chapter 4 Customized Doses Review for Mid-Term Examination	
10	Mid-Term Examination	

Course Schedule
Second 10 Weeks

Week	Topic	Homework Assignment
1	Chapter 5 Household Measure, Oral Doses, Temperature	
2	Chapter 6 Parenteral Injections and Infusions	
3	Chapter 6 Other Units of Measure, Using Powdered Medication	
4	Chapter 7 Percentage and Ratio Strength Dilutions	
5	Chapter 7 IV Flow Rates, Drop Factor and Infusion Rates	
6	Chapter 8 Compounded Formulas, Alligations	
7	Chapter 8 Weight-in-Weight (w/w) Calculations, Special Dilutions	
8	Chapter 9 Business Math, Insurance Reimbursement	
9	Chapter 9 Inventory Review for Final Examination	
10	Comprehensive Final Examination	

Selecting the Instructional Approach, Resources, and Activities

After the course outcomes, delivery mode, and structure are determined, it is important to plan the main content of the course. This planning includes selecting courseware, identifying resources for English language learners, considering instructional support materials, and reviewing supplemental resources.

Student Courseware

Selecting high-quality student courseware is an important step in the planning process. Learning materials should be engaging and accessible. Paradigm Publishing's *Pharmacy Calculations for Technicians* product includes several valuable learning tools to support the course performance objectives.

- *Pharmacy Calculations for Technicians, Fifth Edition* textbook
- Study Partner CD
- Student Internet Resource Center at www.paradigmcollege.net/pharmcalc5e

Textbook

Pharmacy Calculations for Technicians is designed to help students master the types of calculations they must perform as pharmacy technicians within a context of safety and efficiency. Key features of the textbook include the following items:

- **Learning Objectives**, establishing clear goals to focus chapter study
- **Key Terms**, highlighting (in boldface) and defining important vocabulary in the study of pharmacy calculations
- **Body System Icons**, establishing connections between certain medications and the body systems that they are prescribed to treat
- **Marginalia Tips**, providing general math rules, calculation strategies, safety concerns, and other important information that students must be aware of when performing pharmacy calculations and handling medications

  Math Morsels, general math tips

  For Good Measure, hints and rules to remember when performing pharmacy calculations

  Safety in Numbers, safety concerns when working with numbers

  Name Exchange, generic and brand names of frequently dispensed medications

  Put Down Roots, analysis of the word parts of certain math terms

- **Canadian Flag Icon**, indicating content that varies in Canadian pharmacy practice and directing students to explore the Internet Resource Center's Canadian supplement
- **Photos, Figures, Tables**, visually reinforcing the information taught in the chapter
- **Chapter Summary**, providing an overview of the key points of the chapter
- **Key Terms**, offering a compilation of all of the key terms and their definitions in the chapter

- **Assessing Comprehension**, providing 10 multiple-choice questions that cover important chapter concepts
- **Finding Solutions**, presenting 2–4 real-world scenarios to help students gain practice in handling challenging workplace situations
- **Sampling the Certification Exam**, offering students practice for the Certification Exam using questions that have been patterned after the test format
- **Appendices**, providing answer keys for problem sets, additional practice with fractions and percents, common pharmacy abbreviations and acronyms, and a measures and conversions chart
- **Glossary**, offering an alphabetical list of the key terms from the entire textbook

Study Partner CD

Available with each textbook, the Study Partner CD provides several features to help support student learning. Chapter Resources include:

- **Chapter Terms**, providing the key terms and definitions from the chapter with audio support and images
- **Flash Cards**, allowing students to learn key concepts from the chapter in a fun, interactive way
- **Matching**, testing students recall of important content from the chapter
- **Quizzing**, providing students with additional assessment on chapter topics in both practice and reported modes
- **Internet Resource Center link**, directing students to online resources for the textbook

Pharmacy Calculations for Technicians Internet Resource Center

Valuable information for both instructors and students can be found on the *Pharmacy Calculations for Technicians* Internet Resource Center at www.paradigmcollege.net/pharmcalc5e. For students, the Internet Resource Center includes additional information and learning tools, such as handouts, supplemental resources, and links to pharmacy-related topics and organizations.

Resources for English Language Learners[1]

One of the fastest-growing groups of students in higher education is comprised of students whose first language is not English and whose English is not yet equivalent to that of native English speakers in lexicon and syntax. The wide differences in fluency among limited-English speakers make planning for meeting their needs somewhat more complex—and very important.

Chances are that you already know you will have some students whose language skills are not up to the level you expect or want. What? You're not the ELL instructor? Not your job? Think again. Your job is to help *all* the students in your course meet the intended outcomes. So plan how you're going to do this for your limited-English speakers. Begin by assessing early on the language abilities of your students. Try these measures:

- One method is a "one-minute preview." Tear some sheets of paper into four parts and give each student a piece. Ask them no more than two questions and give them one minute (okay, two) to write their answers. The question *could* be about their language skills, but it might be better to ask them something else. That way, you get a short writing sample plus information about something else, such as why they are taking the course, something they would like to learn, the types of activities they enjoy, or what they are most worried about in the course. You don't need to be an English teacher to see which students will need help. Use your common sense.

- If your class is small, conduct a discussion early in the course. Make sure you hear each student answer a question or ask one.
- If you are conducting a pretest for the course, include some questions that ask students if they need to improve their English speaking or writing skills.
- Tell students to e-mail you if they think they will need language help or extra exam time for reading assignments or tests.

In addition to the suggestions above, consider whether or not you need to prepare a list of terms for each session or unit that might be troublesome for English language learners. Do you need to have students arrange for tutors to assist with completing the unguided assessments? Do you need to dedicate a session or part of one to instruction on how to prepare the work you expect?

To assist English language learners in meeting the outcomes and objectives of a pharmacy technician course, direct students at the start of your instruction to ELL support programs at your college, local library, or community center. You may also want to recommend the following support websites:

- Duke University's online instruction and resources for ELL learners http://twp.duke.edu/writing-studio/resources/esl-efl-resources
- Online English pronunciation guide for the generic and brand names of drugs http://rxprontopass.com/index.php?page=free_pronunciations
- Purdue University's Online Writing Lab [OWL] http://owl.english.purdue.edu/owl/
- University of North Carolina's online instruction and resources for ELL learners http://writingcenter.unc.edu/resources/esl

Instructor Resources

Pharmacy Calculations for Technicians offers a comprehensive set of supplements to reinforce student learning and to support instructors in every way possible.

Instructor's Guide

In addition to course planning tools and suggested syllabi, the *Instructor's Guide* provides a pretest; chapter-specific teaching objectives; suggested instructional approaches; teaching tips and activities; chapter-related handouts and their answer keys; answer keys for the end-of-chapter exercises and the chapter practice tests; and additional chapter assessments.

Instructor Resources CD

Accompanying each print *Instructor's Guide*, the Instructor Resources CD includes all of the resources from the print *Instructor's Guide* as well as PowerPoint® presentations to enhance lectures and the **EXAM**VIEW® Assessment Suite.

PowerPoint® Presentations

PowerPoint® presentations are available for each chapter and focus on the important concepts discussed in the textbook. Included in each presentation are interactive content questions to challenge student learning.

EXAMVIEW® Assessment Suite and Test Banks

The **EXAM**VIEW® Assessment Suite is a full-featured, computerized test generator that offers instructors a wide variety of options for generating both print and online tests. The test banks for *Pharmacy Calculations for Technicians* provide 40 questions for each chapter including multiple-choice, true/false, matching, and calculation problems. If the provided bank of items doesn't perfectly meet your needs, the program allows you to add an unlimited number of your own items or edit existing items. You can select new or existing items to create an unlimited number of chapter quizzes, tests, and exams. Using the **EXAM**VIEW® program, you can deliver tests on the Web, on your local area network, or in print.

Pharmacy Calculations for Technicians Internet Resource Center

As mentioned earlier, the Internet Resource Center offers valuable information for both students and instructors. Resources for instructors are available on the password-protected Instructor site and include some of the files found on the Instructor Resources CD (the print *Instructor's Guide* and the PowerPoint® presentations for the textbook chapters). Instructors will also find handouts; supplemental resources; links to pharmacy-related topics and organizations; and a listing of the ASHP correlations, with references to the corresponding textbook components that fulfill these standards.

Distance-Learning Files

Distance-learning files that can be used in a variety of course management platforms—such as Webcourses, Desire 2 Learn, Angel, Moodle, and others—provide materials that allow you to create a customized Web component for your course. Here are ideas for using some of the common course management system tools to their best advantage.

- **Discussion Board.** The discussion board provides an opportunity for every student to interact and become an active learner by posting answers to the weekly discussion question and responding to other students' postings.

- **Assignment Tool.** The assignment tool provides an opportunity for students to upload their homework assignment and have the instructor grade and return either a corrected copy of the assignment or post the corrected solution so students can compare their answers with the corrected solution.

- **Web Streaming.** The latest technology enables the instructor to use Web streaming to introduce each weekly topic and provide additional instruction and guidance to students. Web streaming can help auditory learners who enjoy both reading the material in the textbook and listening to an instructor's lecture.

- **Chat Room.** Chat rooms can provide a nonsynchronized forum for students and can also allow both the instructor and other students to interact in real time.

- **Assessment Tool.** The test bank can be uploaded into the assessment tool so that students can take their quizzes and exams entirely online. One popular technique for creating unique exams is to use the odd-numbered questions from the test bank for creating randomly generated quizzes while saving the even-numbered questions for creating exams and finals.

- **Web Links.** Online courses also provide an opportunity for students to conduct information searches on the Internet and submit research papers as part of their course grade. The instructor can post links to websites such as the Institute for Safe Medication Practices for students to peruse and answer questions on some of the latest issues in relation to avoiding medication errors.

- **Podcasts and Videos.** A variety of course management platforms offer the ability to upload podcast and video files for instructional use.

Professional Support

Instructors may find valuable information, tools, and support from a number of professional pharmacy organizations as well. Two of the most relevant and helpful websites for instructors are those of the American Society of Health-Systems Pharmacists (ASHP) and the Pharmacy Technician Educators Council (PTEC). The ASHP website (http://www.ashp.org) contains the *Model Curriculum for Pharmacy Technician Training, 2nd Edition* information on pursuing ASHP accreditation, and numerous other resources. The PTEC website (http://www.pharmacytecheducators.com) offers resources, pharmacy technician advocacy, pharmacy technician education best practice models, and an opportunity to connect with other pharmacy technician educators.

Developing an Assessment Strategy

The final major phase of planning a course is to develop an assessment strategy based on the purpose of evaluation and on your philosophy of what constitutes high-quality assessments. The obvious purpose of assessing students' learning is to determine whether or not students have achieved the goals of the course and, if they have, to what degree, resulting in a grade for credits earned. Other functions of evaluation include motivating students, determining the overall effectiveness of your teaching, and meeting accreditation requirements.

What is your philosophy of assessment? In shaping one, consider these suggestions from Paradigm Publishing's *Exceptional Teaching*:

1. Assessment should contribute to students' learning by asking them to apply their skills in out-of-school or workplace situations.
2. Timing, content, and form of assessments should be planned as an integral part of the course design.
3. The purpose of every assessment should be clear.
4. The type of assessment—its content and format—should be appropriate for the purpose.
5. Assessments should be scored as consistently and objectively as possible.
6. Assessments should provide students with feedback on their learning.
7. Assessments should emphasize intellectual traits of value: analytical reading, thinking, decision making, and research skills, along with individual creativity and individual intelligence.
8. Assessments should be conducted at specific, planned checkpoints.
9. Assessments should be conducted in a positive learning environment, with every effort made to lower students' test anxieties.
10. Assessments should allow students to demonstrate their accomplishment of outcomes in various ways, including ways that fit their individual learning styles.

Determining the Number, Level, and Type of Assessments

Using your philosophy of assessment as a guide, begin to formulate your evaluation and grading strategy by answering these course-level questions, as presented in *Exceptional Teaching*:

- Do I want a course pre-assessment?
- Do I want a course comprehensive assessment—one that will determine students' mastery of the major intended outcomes for the entire course?
- Do I want pre-assessments for each section or program?
- Do I want comprehensive assessments for each section or program—ones that assess students' mastery of the major intended outcomes for that program?
- Do I want interim or checkpoint assessments that assess students' mastery of intended outcomes of learning chunks within units? How many? How often?
- Once my system is in place, will my students know that I value *how* and *how well* they think?

The questions above will help you establish approximately how many assessments you wish to include and their place in the course. The next decisions concern which types of assessment to use: traditional cognitive (objective) tests and/or performance-based assessments. Each of these two major categories of tests has its best uses. Traditional cognitive tests such as multiple-choice exams usually work best for testing information recall, comprehension, and analysis. They also are reliable and efficient, and relatively easy to score. On the down side, objective-type tests are criticized for not representing how students will use their new skills in an unfamiliar setting or in the real world of work. Here's where performance-based testing rises to the fore. Requiring students to demonstrate what they have learned and to apply it in a realistic context that closely approximates an on-the-job situation measures how well students can do what the course intended to teach them. As emphasized in *Exceptional Teaching*, "Authentic, performance-based assessments ask students to integrate what they have learned and apply it to resolve an issue, solve a problem, create something new, work collaboratively, or use their written and oral communication skills. Authentic assessments stress the process of learning as well as the outcomes of learning."

Typically, instructors develop an assessment strategy that uses the strengths of both major types of assessments, and the assessment resources developed to support *Pharmacy Calculations for Technicians* provide ample opportunity for both objective-based and performance-based assessments.

- The Problem Sets that follow the textbook sections offer performance-based assessments that gauge student comprehension of the section content and student readiness to move to the next skill set.
- The Assessing Comprehension section is an objective-based assessment, offering 10 multiple-choice questions to test students' recall and comprehension of chapter content.
- The Finding Solutions section is a performance-based assessment in which students are presented with real-world scenarios that require them to apply their knowledge to form responses.

- The Sampling the Certification Exam section is an objective-based assessment that prepares students for certification by offering 5 multiple-choice questions modeled after those on the certification examination.

In addition to these textbook assessments, the Study Partner CD and the **EXAM**VIEW® Assessment Suite on the Instructor Resources CD offer additional objective-based and performance-based assessments for students. Lastly, additional, performance-based assessments for each chapter are included in the Additional Assessments and Answer Keys section of this *Instructor's Guide*.

Creating a Grading Plan

By choosing the types of assessments that will measure students' achievement of course and program outcomes, you will already have established a schema of the major grading components. The next step is to weight the scores as preparation for entering them into a grade calculation system, for example, an Excel spreadsheet.

Will you include nonachievement factors, such as effort and attendance, in students' grades? If so, consider how to measure those elements. While it is simple to track attendance, it is not so easy to objectively evaluate effort and attitude. Some experts recommend that teachers provide regular verbal and written feedback on nonachievement factors but confine grades to academic achievement.

Student Textbook Updates

As a service to both instructors and students, and in the interest of instructor and student (and, consequently, patient) safety, Paradigm Publishing provides updates, notes, and corrections related to the content of the student textbook. Some of these changes may include the introduction or removal of drugs by manufacturers or regulating bodies, important changes or amendments to pharmacy standards or laws, additional safety concerns, or corrections to the current student textbook edition. To that end, students and instructors will find these updates on the *Pharmacy Calculations for Technicians* Internet Resource Center in the folder titled "Chapter Resources" and then in a subfolder titled "Chapter Updates." These updates can also be found within the individual chapter folders.

For More Information

Much of the content of this "Planning the Course" section is based on information found in *Exceptional Teaching: Ideas in Action*. To order a copy of this resource, please visit www.emcp.com or call or e-mail Customer Service at 800-535-6865, educate@emcp.com.

Pharmacy Calculations Pretest

A pretest is an important tool for an instructor in a pharmacy calculations course. This test typically covers fractions, decimals, ratios, and percentages and gives instructors a baseline to assess each student's math skills and number sense. As you know, your classroom is comprised of students with varying math backgrounds. Gauging their math abilities allows you to plan your lessons and your class time accordingly. Certain groups of students may remember how to use fractions and decimals and cruise through the first few chapters of the book. Other groups of students may need extra time devoted to a review of basic math skills to build confidence in their problem-solving abilities. A pretest will quickly identify students who fall into the latter group.

A pretest such as the one that follows should be given the first day of class. When administering the test, allow students as much time as they need to complete the assessment. Ask them to place a mark next to the questions that they have no idea how to solve and to skip over those questions until they have completed the remainder of the test. Then tell students to go back to those skipped questions to see if they have gained any insight on solving these problems by working through other questions. Allow students to use a calculator to take the test. Doing so alleviates some of the stress that comes with testing. Calculators are used in the workplace and in everyday life. Using them during class, homework, and tests is common practice and should not be discouraged. To that end, specific questions in the pretest are marked with an asterisk if a calculator is recommended for use during the calculation process.

When students are finished with the pretest, grade the test together and have students grade their own tests. Ask students to put away all of their writing utensils; then provide them with markers or pens of a particular color such as green, blue, or purple. Using designated pen colors is an easy way of maintaining the academic integrity of the pretest (or any test you grade in class with students) while helping students see exactly what they did right and wrong on their tests. It is a good idea to have several sets of "grading markers" available and trade out which color you use on different days.

Pretest

This pretest is being used as a tool for your instructor in order to help determine what math skills you have. The test covers fractions, decimals, ratios, and percentages. It will be graded, but your score will be based on taking the test, not on how many you get right or wrong.

Identify the fraction with the largest value.

1. ⅙   ⅛

2. ⅔   ⅞

Identify the fraction with the smallest value.

3. $\frac{1}{10}$ $\frac{1}{100}$

4. ⅗ $\frac{5}{3}$

Reduce the following fractions to their lowest value.

5. $\frac{4}{12}$

6. $\frac{15}{36}$

Perform the following calculations with fractions and reduce the answers to their lowest values.

7. ⅓ + ½ =

8. $\frac{4}{7} - \frac{1}{7}$ =

Convert the following ratios to decimal values.

9. 3:4

10. 1:100

Solve the following story problems.

11. Jane has 12 deck chairs and she has painted ¼ of them yellow. How many are unpainted?

12. Taking a shower uses ½ of the water that a bath requires in the Smith home. If a bath requires 8 gallons, how much water does a shower use?

13. One out of every five tablets in Greg's medication container is broken. If the container has 100 tablets in it, how many tablets are broken?

14. Susan is making two batches of cookies. Her first batch will use a recipe that calls for ⅓ cup of sugar. The second batch will use a recipe that calls for ¾ cup of sugar. How many cups of sugar will be used to make the two batches of cookies?

*15. What is the price of an item that is $16.99 and is marked 25% off?

*16. The electric bill is 30% higher than this time last year. If the bill was $154.90 one year ago, what is it now?

*17. Samantha only watches 6 of the 200 channels available to her on cable TV. What percentage of the total number of channels does she watch?

*18. The Excedrin Migraine label states that the box contains an additional 20% "free." If the regular-sized box has 100 tablets, how many extra tablets are included?

*19. A bottle containing 150 mL is dispensed for a child who uses 5 mL, three times daily. How long will this bottle last?

*20. Jason's paycheck is $410.34 before taxes and other deductions. How much does he make per hour if he worked 38.5 hours in this pay period?

---

* The use of a calculator is recommended to solve this problem.

21. If the selling price of a product is $7.99 and the pharmacy cost is $4.05, how much profit in dollars does the pharmacy make on the sale?

*22. If a pharmacy needs to mark up a product that costs $2.30 by 40%, what will the selling price be?

*23. If a prescription drug is marked up 20% and the cost for the pharmacy is $46.75, what will the selling price be?

*24. An inhaler has 200 inhalations in it. The patient uses 2 inhalations three times daily. How many days will it last?

25. A pharmacy charges $45.49 for a prescription. If a patient has to pay 20% and the insurance pays 80% of the cost of the medication, how much will the patient have to pay?

---

* The use of a calculator is recommended to solve this problem.

Pretest Answer Key

1. $\frac{1}{6}$
2. $\frac{7}{8}$
3. $\frac{1}{100}$
4. $\frac{3}{5}$
5. $\frac{1}{3}$
6. $\frac{5}{12}$
7. Since $\frac{1}{3} = \frac{2}{6}$ and $\frac{1}{2} = \frac{3}{6}$, $\frac{2}{6} + \frac{3}{6} = \frac{5}{6}$
8. $\frac{4}{7} - \frac{1}{7} = \frac{3}{7}$
9. $\frac{3}{4} = 0.75$
10. $\frac{1}{100} = 0.01$
11. $\frac{4}{4}$ total chairs − $\frac{1}{4}$ painted chairs = $\frac{3}{4}$ unpainted chairs; $\frac{3}{4}$ unpainted chairs × 12 chairs = 9 unpainted chairs
12. $\frac{1}{2}$ bath × 8 gallons/bath = 4 gallons
13. $\frac{1}{5}$ tablets × 100 tablets = 20 tablets that are broken
14. $\frac{1}{3} = \frac{4}{12}$ and $\frac{3}{4} = \frac{9}{12}$; $\frac{4}{12} + \frac{9}{12} = \frac{13}{12}$ cups, or $1\frac{1}{12}$ cups
15. \$16.99 × 0.25 = \$4.25; \$16.99 − 4.25 = \$12.74
16. \$154.90 × 0.3 = \$46.47; \$154.90 + \$46.47 = \$201.37
17. $\frac{6}{200} = 0.03$; 0.03 × 100 = 3%
18. 100 tablets × 20% (or 0.20) = 20 free tablets
19. 5 mL/dose × 3 doses/day = 15 mL/day; 150 mL /15 mL/day = 10 days
20. \$410.34 pay/38.5 hours = \$10.66 pay/ per hour
21. \$7.99 − \$4.05 = \$3.94
22. 40% = 0.4; \$2.30 × 0.4 = \$0.92; and \$2.30 + \$0.92 = \$3.22
23. 20% = 0.2; \$46.75 × 0.2 = \$9.35; \$46.75 + \$9.35 = \$56.10
24. 2 inhalations/dose × 3 doses/day = 6 inhalations/day; 200 inhalations per vial / 6 inhalations per day = 33.33 days per vial, rounded to 33 days per vial
25. \$45.49 × 20% (or 0.20) = \$9.098, rounded to \$9.10

Chapter Lessons

As an instructor, you know that lesson preparation is essential to providing the best learning environment for your students. This preparation involves knowing the chapter content, understanding the needs of your learners, and varying your instructional approaches. Teaching math presents an additional challenge to instructors: breaking down the barriers that prevent math-phobic students from achieving success in your classroom.

This introduction provides some general guidelines and suggestions for teaching a pharmacy calculations course. This section also offers explanations regarding some of the different instructional approaches for teaching math. Read through these topics carefully for many of them relate to areas that students often struggle to understand. This general preparation section is followed by chapter-specific suggestions to help you in the planning of your course.

Course Organization

Prior to teaching a pharmacy calculations course, be sure to consider how you want to structure your class time and what supplies are necessary for effective instruction.

Suggested Class Structure

When teaching mathematics, establishing a consistent class structure helps both students and instructors manage their class time. Table 1 lists a suggested schedule for a 90-minute pharmacy calculations class. The suggested times can be adjusted as needed to correspond with your class length. When planning the course, be sure to allow students time to take a mental and physical break, as well as time to ask questions.

Table 1: Suggested Schedule for a 90-Minute Pharmacy Calculations Class

Allotted Time	Activity
10 minutes	Homework discussion; response to questions
15 minutes	Quiz
10 minutes	Review of concepts
5 minutes	Break
30 minutes	Presentation of new material
15 minutes	Review and complete in-class practice problems
5 minutes	Assign homework for next session and answer student questions

Start each day with a 10-minute review of the topic covered in the previous class session; then collect homework and respond to questions about the homework assignment. A follow-up 15-minute quiz comprised of five or fewer questions provides you with a snapshot of your students' comprehension of previously presented material. Consider using an audience response system such as iClicker or polleverywhere.com to immediately assess student quizzes. Then spend 10 minutes reviewing the math concepts from the previous lesson, focusing particular attention on the types of questions that students struggled with during the quiz. At this point, giving students a 5-minute break from numbers and calculations allows them to recharge before launching into the next lesson. Allot about 30 minutes to present the new material, followed by a 15-minute review and in-class practice problems. Finally, use the last 5 minutes of class to give students their homework assignment and answer any remaining questions.

Remember that math concepts often work as building blocks, so it is important to evaluate and return homework assignments and quizzes promptly to help you assess student understanding of the material. Conducting weekly student assessments helps you detect students who are falling behind their peers.

Instructional Approaches

Prior to teaching a pharmacy calculations course, be sure to consider procedures that you want to establish on note taking, group work, and quizzing. These procedures help to establish your class structure and should be made clear to your students at the start of your course.

Note Taking

Students at this level of mathematical study need guided notes that will assist them in working through the material independently after class. Encourage students to take detailed notes as example calculations are demonstrated in class. Suggested techniques for note taking for a math class are listed in Table 2. Discuss these tips with students, many of whom have no idea how to take notes in a math class.

Table 2: Tips for Taking Notes in a Math Class

- Use a pencil with a good eraser to take notes.
- Take your notes on lined notebook paper to keep your notes neat and legible.
- Take notes only on one side of the paper, and number the pages so that the material stays in order.
- Stay alert.
- Write down questions or key terminology and phrases presented by the instructor.
- Leave plenty of space between each problem and in the margins. Use the margins for supplementary notes when you review the material at home.
- Write out each calculation step, and do not skip steps.
- Label all numbers with the proper units.
- Do not jump ahead to work on homework assignments during class presentations.
- Ideally, try to review notes within 24 hours or sooner, if possible. Revise your notes as needed for clarity.

Taking detailed notes and writing out each step can be invaluable for students when they review notes at home. It is helpful to use the examples in the text by writing them on the overhead or board. You may also want to share other examples that you have prepared for class to give students added practice. Be sure to allow time for students to work on these examples in class and ask any questions as they work through the calculations. Then present the solutions to these problems and invite any additional questions.

Group Work

Devoting a portion of class time for group problem solving offers many benefits for students. Struggling students can talk through the calculation steps with others and ask questions in a small-group setting. Math-savvy students can serve as peer helpers and can lead the group discussion. All students can learn that math can be approached in several ways—all of which can be valid methods for solving a problem. For some general guidelines on group work in math class, see Table 3 below.

Table 3: Using Groups in Math Class

- Establish groups of 4–6 students. Be sure that each group has 1–2 students who are proficient in math. Reassign groups each week as needed.
- Present your examples to the class and then assign each group a problem.
- Have the group members work on their problem together and come to a consensus as to the correct answer.
- Ask one representative from each group to write the solution out on the board and explain it to the class. Be sure that this task is shared by all group members at some point.
- Collect each group's final answers to document student participation in class and to assign grades.
- Monitor groups for participation from all students.
- Allow time at the end of each class for groups to get started on homework.

Quizzing

Monitor student understanding of the math concepts by implementing frequent, short quizzes. Many instructors find that providing a short quiz each class period helps students overcome math anxiety as well as test anxiety. Each quiz should include a range of pharmacy calculation problems, from easy problems requiring simple conversions to challenging problems needing complex calculations. There are advantages to giving the quiz at the beginning of class and at the end of class. Giving the quiz early in the class period allows students to tackle review work first, thus giving students a better focus on new material when it is presented. Starting class with a quiz also alleviates the mounting test anxiety that comes with giving the quiz at the end of class. On the other hand, giving the quiz at the end of the class period gives students the chance to raise questions about homework assignments, allowing you the opportunity to assess the readiness of students to take the quiz. If students are hesitant and do not fully grasp the material, quizzing at the end of class may work well. This will allow time for a more adequate review leading up to the quiz.

Incorporating technological components such as an anonymous audience response system offers several advantages: For students, using this type of technology allows for interactive learning and transforms the anxiety-filled test experience into something that is engaging and fun; for instructors, the use of an audience response system provides immediate feedback as to whether or not students have grasped the day's material. Some of the more commonly used audience response systems are iClicker and polleverywhere.com.

General Supplies

To teach a pharmacy calculations course, be sure that your classroom has the basic supplies listed below. Specific supplies that you will need for a particular chapter can be found in the individual chapter lesson section.

- Dry-erase markers for the whiteboard or chalk for the blackboard
- Markers for overhead transparencies
- Paper for practicing math problems in groups
- A set of simple calculators (to ensure preprogrammed calculators are not used to cheat)*
- Pencils and erasers
- A minimum of three sets of colored pens or markers to use for grading in class (to avoid student tampering during in-class grading)

    Note: You will need to determine the class policy for the use of calculators. Be aware that simple calculators are allowed when students take the Pharmacy Technician Certification Examination (PTCE), and calculators are commonplace in the work environment. Electronic calculation offers advantages of speed and accuracy, provided students enter the data correctly.

Content Preparation

Effective pharmacy calculations instructors understand that engaging students requires extensive content preparation, an understanding of math pedagogy, and the use of multiple supplemental resources. These factors are important to student engagement and success in the classroom.

Student Textbook

When planning your course, spend time familiarizing yourself with the structure of the textbook and the individual chapters, as well as the math approaches demonstrated in the instructions and examples.

Chapter Organization

Every chapter in *Pharmacy Calculations for Technicians, Fifth Edition* is divided into sections, each designed to introduce one or more specific mathematical concepts. The corresponding problem sets apply these concepts and are designed to take approximately one hour of time to complete, once the material is understood by the student.

Use the students' pretest scores to determine their approach to the chapter content. For those students who scored above average on the pretest, encourage them to read the chapter and work out some or all of the problems in the problem sets before class so that they are familiar with the concepts before the calculations are demonstrated in class. For students whose pretest scores were average or below average, recommend that they *only* read the chapter and not practice any problems until they build some confidence in their math abilities. For these students, your step-by-step guidance and positive feedback during the calculation process ensure that the math procedures are learned correctly—and you build on that progress rather than spend time "unteaching" or "reteaching" math concepts.

Make sure students are confident in completing the calculations in one section before moving on to the next section because many of the concepts and skills build on each other. Do not proceed until a majority of students demonstrate their understanding of the content. If an individual student is falling behind, make arrangements for the student to meet with you during office hours to discuss his or her challenges with the material.

Body System Icons

Body system icons accompany the names of generic and brand name medications to assist students in connecting the medications with the body systems they are prescribed to treat. This feature is not intended to be a primary teaching tool in this textbook. Rather, students should learn pharmacology using a textbook written for that purpose, such as Paradigm Publishing's *Pharmacology for Technicians, Fifth Edition*. Although many of the medications discussed in the textbook are used on multiple systems, the body system icons chosen fit the contexts of the drug dosages or sigs used in the examples. Consequently, explain to students that a particular drug may have a Nervous System icon in one section but a Pain and Pyrexia icon in another section. To illustrate this scenario, refer to Table 4 below that shows the different applications of diphenhydramine and furosemide.

Table 4: Applications of Body System Icons

Medication	Dosage Form	Indication	Body System	Example
Diphenhydramine (Benadryl)	Tablets	Induce sleep at bedtime	Nervous System	R̞ **Diphenhydramine XXV mg** Sig: ii tab each night Disp: XXXII tablets
	Capsules	Relieve itching	Nervous System and Integumentary System	R̞ **Diphenhydramine capsules** ii cap po qid prn itching
	Elixir	Relieves itching in a pediatric patient	Integumentary System	NDC 0000-0000-00 **4 fl oz** **Diphenhydramine** Hydrochloride Elixir USP **12.5 mg/5 mL** R$_x$ only

Medication	Dosage Form	Indication	Body System	Example
	Elixir	Reduces inflammation in the lungs, relieves itching, prevents system release of histamine due to allergy	Respiratory System and Nervous System	NDC 0000-0000-00 4 fl oz **Diphenhydramine** Hydrochloride Elixir USP **12.5 mg/5 mL** R_x only
Furosemide (Lasix)	Tablet	Reduces edema	Urinary System	Lasix 20 mg; take 1 tab QD in AM for edema
	Injection	Reduces edema, improves cardiac function	Urinary System and Cardiovascular System	NDC 63323-280-02 28002 **FUROSEMIDE** INJECTION, USP 20 mg/2 mL (10 mg/mL) For IM or IV Use Rx only **2 mL** Single Dose Vial Preservative Free Discard unused portion. **PROTECT FROM LIGHT.** APP Pharmaceuticals, LLC Schaumburg, IL 60173 401803D LOT/EXP 63323-280-02 Sample label. Please see package insert for complete prescribing information. Images used with permission from Fresenius Kabi USA, LLC

Math Pedagogy

When teaching pharmacy calculations, instructors and students should be aware that there are several ways to set up equations in order to solve math problems. As long as the equations are mathematically sound, the setup of the problem or the calculation method used may vary.

Calculation Methods

The most commonly used pharmacy calculation methods include ratio and proportion and dimensional analysis. Both methods are used in this textbook.

Ratio and Proportion Method When using ratio-proportion, the *x* is used to signify the unknown variable, or the unknown quantity that must be determined through the problem-solving process. Note that the *x* may be placed in different locations in the equation, depending on the setup that the instructor or student prefers. Regardless of the position of the variable, the steps for solving the problem using cancellation or cross multiplication are the same. Still, providing a consistent equation setup—for example, always placing the *x* in a ratio in the same position when creating a proportion—helps to avoid confusion for students and allows them to more confidently approach and solve the problem.

To demonstrate two different equation setups for a ratio-proportion problem, refer to the following problems and solutions:

Problem

Calculate how many milliliters of furosemide are needed to fill a prescription order of 60 mg. You have on hand a solution containing 10 mg/mL.

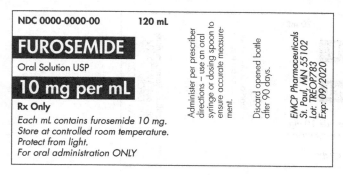

Solution A

1. Set up the equation and place the x in the upper left location.

$$\frac{x \text{ mL furosemide}}{60 \text{ mg}} = \frac{1 \text{ mL furosemide}}{10 \text{ mg}}$$

2. Multiply both sides of the equation by 60 mg.

$$\frac{(60 \text{ mg}) \, x \text{ mL furosemide}}{60 \text{ mg}} = \frac{1 \text{ mL furosemide } (60 \text{ mg})}{10 \text{ mg}}$$

3. Cancel out 60 mg and solve for x.

$$\frac{(\cancel{60 \text{ mg}}) \, x \text{ mL furosemide}}{\cancel{60 \text{ mg}}} = \frac{1 \text{ mL furosemide } (60 \text{ mg})}{10 \text{ mg}}$$

$$x \text{ mL furosemide} = \frac{1 \text{ mL } (60 \text{ mg})}{10 \text{ mg}}$$

$$x \text{ mL} = 6 \text{ mL}$$

Solution B

1. Place the x in the lower right location and use cross multiplication.

$$\frac{x \text{ mL furosemide}}{60 \text{ mg}} = \frac{1 \text{ mL furosemide}}{10 \text{ mg}}$$

2. Cross multiply.

$$1 \times 60 = 60; \ 60/10 = 6$$

$$x \text{ mL} = 6 \text{ mL}$$

Dimensional Analysis Method When using dimensional analysis, place the unknown variable (*x*) by itself.

Problem

Calculate how many milliliters of furosemide are needed to fill a prescription order of 60 mg. You have on hand a solution containing 10 mg/mL.

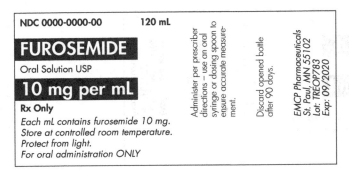

Solution C

1. desired dose × volume of unit/dose in unit = *x*

2. 60 mg × 1 mL/10 mg = *x*

    60/10 = *x*

    x = 6 mL

As you can see, each of these three solutions is correct despite the varying approaches to solving the problem. Stress to students that they should use their preferred method when solving pharmacy calculation problems—in other words, they should choose a method that instills the greatest level of confidence in their work. Examples in the student textbook reflect several different approaches for setting up conversions and solutions.

Showing Work

You will note that the "work" of how to solve problems is shown in its entirety in Chapters 1–3 of the textbook and wanes with the subsequent chapters. By the time that students are studying Chapter 4, they should know how to solve for *x* using either the ratio-proportion method or the dimensional analysis method without being led through each step. It is important to show every step in your calculation process when working problems on the board. Most students need that visual reminder as they are learning new mathematical concepts. Mention to students that, in practice, experienced pharmacy personnel often get to the point where certain steps may be eliminated because they are done from rote memory. Students should be instructed to do whatever they need to do to be confident that their calculations are 100% accurate. Remind students that they should always double-check their own calculations prior to filling a prescription or otherwise preparing a medication.

Rounding Numbers

Rounding numbers and determining when and where to round are skills that pharmacists and pharmacy technicians learn with experience. Math rounding procedures vary among pharmacy practice settings. For example, some facilities have an established policy to always round to the tenth; other pharmacies may implement a policy that dictates rounding to the hundredth. Still other facilities may always round down in certain situations. In practice, be sure to refer to your facility's Policy and Procedure (P&P) manual for specific rounding rules.

Rounding Adult Dosages

A general rule to follow is to round to the closest degree of precision that is measurable given the dosage type and measuring instrument that is used. For example, when calculating a dosage that is to be administered via an oral syringe, the dose should be rounded to the nearest amount that an oral syringe is capable of accurately measuring. For an oral syringe, that amount is likely a tenth of a milliliter. In general, when calculating and measuring an injectable drug dosage, the use of sterile parenteral syringes are more highly calibrated, allowing for relatively easy measurement of volumes to the tenth or even hundredth of a milliliter.

The approach taken in the textbook is to round to the nearest hundredth unless otherwise indicated. Students struggle with knowing when it is appropriate to round to what decimal point. So while they are learning the math procedures, suggest to them that they always round to the same place at the final calculation. Once they are confident in their ability to identify situations where they need to round to a different decimal value, direct them to do so.

Some instructors prefer that students round to the tenth and—if this is the case—simply advise the students of your expectations. In most cases, the answer key is rounded to the hundredths place, so adjust the answer that you accept accordingly. Keep in mind that students who have learned dosage calculations using a nursing textbook are often in the practice of rounding to the tenth in all situations.

Rounding Pediatric Dosages

Pediatric dosages, especially when a patient is less than one year old or under a certain identified weight, are generally rounded down. Pediatric patients are more likely to experience side effects and adverse reactions to medications, and a very slight dosage change may be the difference between safe and dangerous doses. Hospital facilities have differing policies about when to round down for these patients. Pediatric doses will typically be measured to the hundredths place. It is important for instructors to be aware of regional and specific institutional practices, so that students are aware of the requirements. Be sure to remind students that in practice they must refer to their facility's P&P manual for pediatric rounding procedures.

Rounding Dollar Amounts

When rounding dollar amounts, it is common practice to round to the nearest cent, at the end of the calculations. For example, the cost of a medication per pill may be $1.348 per tablet, but the cost will not be rounded until the final calculation.

Supplemental Resources

In addition to the print *Instructor's Guide*, be sure to incorporate the Study Partner CD as well as the Internet Resource Center in your course planning.

Study Partner CD

The Study Partner CD, which accompanies every student textbook, offers key terms review, matching activities, interactive flash cards, and practice quizzes. This CD may be used for independent student practice, assigned homework exercises, or required assessment of skills. For the latter category, each chapter offers a multiple-choice quiz that is available in both Practice and Reported modes. In the Practice mode, students receive immediate feedback on each quiz item and a report of his or her total score. On-screen feedback references the numbered section in which the calculation is taught in the chapter. In the Reported mode, the results are e-mailed to both the instructor and the student. With that in mind, you may choose to use the quizzes as part of an in-class review of the calculations taught in a chapter, as a homework assignment, or as a graded exam.

Internet Resource Center

The Internet Resource Center (IRC) provides a wealth of material for both students and instructors. For students, the IRC allows them to access key terms, handouts, and assessments for the course. They can also find supplemental resources online, including the textbook appendices, pharmacy guides, pharmacy safety information, and professional organizations. For instructors, the IRC provides the complete *Instructor's Guide*, as well as ASHP correlations, PowerPoint presentations, textbook image banks, medication labels, and additional handouts that cover the apothecary system. All of these tools are invaluable to instructors while constructing their coursework.

Chapter 1   Understanding Subdivisions of Numbers, Number Systems, Estimating, and Accuracy

Set Your Purpose

Upon completion of this chapter, you should ensure that students are able to meet the following learning objectives:

- Understand fractions and be able to compare them, express them as decimals, and find common denominators.
- Manipulate fractions by adding, subtracting, multiplying, and dividing them.
- Interpret Roman and Arabic numbers and convert values between the two systems.
- Read scientific notation and convert large and small numbers to scientific notation.
- Determine the value of a decimal and accurately round off decimal values.
- Estimate drug doses in order to check the accuracy of final calculations.
- Perform calculations while retaining accuracy and the correct number of significant figures.
- Understand conversions between standard time and 24-hour time.

Preview the Chapter

Chapter 1 reviews numbers with students, including their systems, subdivisions, and basic operations. This chapter also covers the use of estimation and significant figures in the calculation process.

- **Section 1.1: Fractions**
  - covers fractions, including the addition, subtraction, multiplication, and division of fractions; reviews the reduction of fractions
- **Section 1.2: Number Systems**
  - discusses Roman numerals, the Arabic number system, and scientific notation
- **Section 1.3: Decimals**
  - reviews decimal places
  - covers addition, subtraction, multiplication, and division of decimals
  - explains the rounding of decimals
- **Section 1.4: Estimates**
  - explains the estimation of sums and the estimation of drug doses
- **Section 1.5: Significant Figures and Measurement Accuracy**
  - demonstrates the counting of significant figures
  - explains the accuracy of significant figures
- **Section 1.6: Time of Day**
  - compares standard time with military or 24-hour time

Plan Ahead

Prior to teaching this chapter, consider the following recommendations:

- Turn to the Pretest section and photocopy (or download and print from the Internet Resource Center) the pretest to distribute to your students. This assessment will help you gauge your students' number sense and math skills.
- Turn to the Handouts section and photocopy (or download and print from the Internet Resource Center) the following item for later distribution to students:
  - Chapter 1, Finding Solutions, Scenario D, #9
- Gather the following supplies that you will need to teach this chapter:
  - dry-erase markers for the whiteboard or chalk for the blackboard
  - markers for overhead transparencies
  - paper for practicing math problems in groups
  - a set of simple calculators (to ensure preprogrammed calculators are not used to cheat)
  - pencils and erasers
  - a minimum of three sets of colored pens or markers to use for grading in class (to avoid any student tampering during in-class grading)

- Consider creating games to assist students in learning fractions and decimals. There are a number of free websites that provide math games based on television shows such as *Jeopardy, Wheel of Fortune,* or *Who Wants to be a Millionaire?* Instructors can download these games at the following websites:
  - www.math-play.com
  - www.sharemylesson.com
  - www.quizlet.com
  - www.coolmath-games.com
  - www.softschools.com/math/games
  - www.hand2mind.com

Establish a Context

Many students enter a math course with some trepidation. In fact, fractions are one of the least favorite math subjects for returning students. Providing students with a pretest that allows them to see the practical applications of fractions in pharmacy practice may help alleviate some of their math anxiety. Another way to build confidence among your students is to use a slow, deliberate approach when teaching the math concepts and skills in Chapter 1. Be sure that students master converting fractions to decimals and percentages, grasp place value and the movement of the decimal point, and understand the standard rounding principles.

Expand Your Lesson

The following section provides teaching tips and suggested activities that you may use to supplement your usual coursework instruction. The teaching tips suggest hints, alternative approaches, learning strategies, safety reminders, and outside resources for instructors to use. The suggested activities offer ideas for small-group and large-group discussion, related in-class activities, or homework exercises. As the course instructor, you are encouraged to modify these ideas to fit your teaching style and the needs of your students. Change them as time permits so that you address the multiple learning styles of your students.

Teaching Tips

General Math Tips

- Remind students that the key to the body system icons that accompany the drug names in this chapter can be found on page xvi of the Preface.
- Refer students to Appendix C: Common Pharmacy Abbreviations and Acronyms if they need assistance in interpreting the meanings of abbreviations and acronyms used in the examples.
- Be sure that students have a solid understanding of basic math including working with decimals, fractions, and percents. This is essential for ensuring student success in later chapters that are built upon these basic math principles.
- Use the pretest to determine which of your students might require additional support from you or a designated tutor or learning laboratory.

- Provide students with as many "real-world" examples as possible. They will benefit from reading drug vials and from working with fractions, decimals, and ratios that are based upon these items.
- Explain your preference as an instructor as to when you want students to round their answers.

Fractions and Percentages

- Review the terms commonly used with fractions, such as *numerator, denominator, improper fraction, mixed number, lowest common denominator*, etc.
- Perform fraction manipulation on the board so that students can follow the step-by-step process. Don't skip any steps, even if you think that the step may be too simplistic, easy, or universally understood.
- Review how to find a least common denominator.
- Provide students with examples of how fractions are used in pharmacy practice (e.g., ½ tablet, compounding a batch that is 1½ times the original recipe, etc.).
- Review what percentages (percent = per 100) are and give examples.

Number Systems

- Discuss Roman numerals and explain their use on prescriptions.

Scientific Notation

- Inform students that they should have an understanding of scientific notation as a basic math skill; however, the concept of scientific notation is generally not used in pharmacy calculations.

Decimals

- Discuss place value and decimal notation using Figure 1.3 in the textbook.
- Discuss the relationship between decimals and fractions and the conversion process.

Estimates

- Explain the rationale behind the use of estimation and provide students with examples. Stress that estimates are a means of building confidence in the accuracy of the basic mathematics calculation process.
- Remind students that most estimating is done "in the head." Encourage students to use the estimation process in their approach to all pharmacy calculation problems in subsequent chapters.
- Inform students that they should have an understanding of estimation as a basic math skill; however, the concept of estimation is generally not used in pharmacy calculations.

Significant Figures

- Students have a tendency to get confused by the information related to significant figures. Be prepared to work out multiple examples on the whiteboard and then assign additional problems for small-group and individual student practice.
- Explain significant figures and why they are important when rounding.

- Discuss the pharmacy practice of never using a "trailing" zero (i.e., a zero after the decimal point [1.0]). Trailing zeros are listed on the Institute for Safe Medication Practices' (ISMP's) *List of Error-Prone Abbreviations, Symbols,* and *Dose Designations.*
- Discuss the pharmacy practice of never leaving a "naked" decimal (i.e., a decimal without a number prior to the decimal point [.1]). Naked decimals are also listed on the ISMP's *List of Error-Prone Abbreviations, Symbols,* and *Dose Designations.*

Time of Day
- Review telling time and compare standard time with 24-hour time. Remind students that 24-hour time is often referred to as "military time."

Suggested Activities
- Distribute the Pretest to students prior to presenting the Chapter 1 content. Use the results of this test to help you determine how much additional instruction and practice are needed to cover the math concepts of fractions, decimals, ratios, and percentages presented in Chapters 1 and 2.
- Distribute the Chapter 1 handout to students prior to assigning the end-of-chapter exercises for their completion. Be sure that students use pencils to shade in the correct amount on the dosing spoon.
- Stop frequently during the math skills lessons to provide students with an opportunity to practice what they have just learned. Have students work independently, with a partner, or in a small group.
- As students work in groups or pairs, assign the homework for the chapter and have students begin work on questions if time permits.
- Give a short quiz to assess understanding of the math concepts presented.
- Use the applications at the end of chapter as the quiz or culminating group assignment. Have a student from each group write their solution on the board and explain it.
- Consider incorporating one of the many free games available to help your students learn basic math skills, including working with fractions, decimals, ratios, percents, and conversions between standard and military time.

Chapter 2   Using Ratios, Percents, and Proportions

Set Your Purpose

Upon completion of this chapter, you should ensure that students are able to meet the following learning objectives:
- Describe the use of ratios and proportions in the pharmacy.
- Solve pharmacy calculations by using ratios and proportions.
- Calculate percentage of error in measurements.

Preview the Chapter

Chapter 2 discusses three important math concepts in pharmacy calculations: ratios, percents, and proportions.

- **Section 2.1: Numerical Ratios**
  - covers the different ways ratios are read and written
  - discusses how ratios are used
- **Section 2.2: Percents**
  - explores the relationship of percents and ratios related to drug dose concentration
  - explains the conversions between ratio and percent and decimal
- **Section 2.3: Proportions**
  - discusses the use of ratios and proportions to perform conversions and to solve story problems
- **Section 2.4: Percentage of Error**
  - describes calculation of percentage of error (a skill that is not critical to student success in future chapters)

Plan Ahead

Prior to teaching this chapter, consider the following recommendations:

- Turn to the Handouts section and photocopy (or download and print from the Internet Resource Center) the following item for later distribution to students:
  - Chapter 2, Finding Solutions, Scenario A, #1
- Gather the following supplies that you will need to teach this chapter:
  - dry-erase markers for the whiteboard or chalk for the blackboard
  - markers for overhead transparencies
  - paper for practicing math problems in groups
  - a set of simple calculators (to ensure preprogrammed calculators are not used to cheat)
  - pencils and erasers
  - a minimum of three sets of colored pens or markers to use for grading in class (to avoid any student tampering during in-class grading)
  - measuring devices including graduated cylinders, large-volume syringes, beakers, oral dosing spoons, and amber ovals
  - liquid for measuring volume (e.g., water)
  - several fun-size bags of M&Ms or Skittles and one large (1 lb) bag of M&Ms or Skittles for the proportion activity outlined below

Establish a Context

A discussion of ratios and percents provides students with the perfect opportunity to get away from those fractions that they dislike so much! Converting a fraction into a ratio, decimal, or percent creates a sense of relief for many students and allows them to manipulate the numbers easier. Another benefit of working with percents is that most students have a basic grasp of this math concept from shopping as a consumer. While these students are skilled at doing mental math with basic percentages, many of them will need written practice with percentages that are not so easily calculable.

The first two sections of the chapter, numerical ratios and percents, are important concepts for students to master before moving into the section that discusses proportions. Be sure that students understand the different ways that ratios can be written and still be "true" or valid representations of the numerical relationship.

Once you are confident that students understand the first two sections, proceed to the third section that covers proportions. In this section, tell students that the ratio-proportion method is an essential calculation process that is used in the remaining chapters of the book. Therefore, direct students to Tables 2.2 and 2.3 for an understanding of the basic rules and steps associated with this calculation method and provide them with plenty of opportunities for practice. For example, assign several problems for students to work on in small groups or pairs. Ask the groups to set up the problems but not perform the calculations until you verify their work. Verifying problem setups allows you to monitor students' understanding of the math concepts and reteach as needed, before students have learned incorrect calculation processes.

The last section of this chapter discusses percentage of error. Inform students that this calculation is not typically performed by pharmacy technicians but is a concept that they need to understand. You may also want to reassure students that although it is important to understand the concept of percentage of error, mastery of this particular concept is not critical to their successful understanding of the pharmacy math concepts discussed in upcoming chapters.

Expand Your Lesson

The following section provides teaching tips and suggested activities that you may use to supplement your usual coursework instruction. The teaching tips suggest hints, alternative approaches, learning strategies, safety reminders, and outside resources for instructors to use. The suggested activities offer ideas for small-group and large-group discussion, related in-class activities, or homework exercises. As the course instructor, you are encouraged to modify these ideas to fit your teaching style and the needs of your students. Change them as time permits so that you address the multiple learning styles of your students.

Teaching Tips

General Math Tips
- Remind students that the key to the body system icons that accompany the drug names in this chapter can be found on page xvi of the Preface.
- Refer students to Appendix C: Common Pharmacy Abbreviations and Acronyms if they need assistance in interpreting the meanings of abbreviations and acronyms used in the examples.
- Take the time to work out each problem in your own handwriting, well ahead of time. Be sure to verify your calculations and answers. Consider keeping them in plastic sheet protectors in a three-ring binder so that you can easily:
  - remove the problems and have them in your hand while you are working the problem on the board
  - assist students while they are working out problems

– use the problems as a model for other problems you want to work out on the board.

- Because this chapter introduces detailed story problems, devote some class time to establishing good habits for reading and setting up story problems.

- Be sure to assign adequate practice problems once students have shown a good grasp of the ratio-proportion method; consider having students work problems in small groups and then take turns working the problems out on the board prior to assigning students to work problems individually.

- Be sure to have students record the problems and the step-by-step calculations used to solve the problems so that they can refer to their notes as needed.

- For those problems that you plan on assigning to your students as homework, consider working out the problems using one or two alternative methods. That way, you are acknowledging the validity of using different approaches for students who arrive at their answers using alternative methods.

- Allow students the opportunity to get started on homework problems during class time. That way, you can monitor their understanding of the concepts and can determine any problem areas that require additional instruction.

Numerical Ratios

- Review with students the different ways that fractions are read aloud and written. Tell them that the *ratio in fraction form* is what will be used in this calculations course and that you will refer to this math concept as a *ratio* from this point forward.

- Discuss how to find ratios on drug labels by referring to the labels used in the text.

- Describe good habits for reading and setting up story problems. Tell students to *always*:

  – identify what they are looking for in the story problem and then highlight this information either by circling it or underlining it.

  – write out the units and descriptions of what they are trying to find (for example, x mg of amoxicillin)

  – place the numbers with the units on a stacked ratio (fraction) to solve a story problem

  – rewrite the units when they are writing out the next steps of solving an equation

- Review Tables 2.2 and 2.3 on page 54 of the textbook with your students to ensure their understanding of the ratio-proportion rules and calculation process for solving for x. You may want to have students turn down the corner of the page for easy reference.

Percents

- Discuss the percent examples in the text with your students to clarify understanding.

- Remind students to think of percent as *parts of 100*. In light of that explanation, explain to students that when determining percent strength or solving for percent, the unknown "x" should always be placed above 100 in the ratio.

Proportions

- Introduce proportions as being a comparison of two ratios.

- To clarify the concept of proportions, conduct several hands-on activities such as the one listed below.

Percentage of Error

- Gauge your students' understanding of ratios, percents, and proportions and their level of frustration before proceeding to a discussion of percentage of error. You may want to defer your instruction of this math concept to another class period.

- Review the concepts of means and extremes as a way to verify the accuracy of a calculation.

Suggested Activities

- Distribute the Chapter 2 handout to students prior to assigning the end-of-chapter exercises. Be sure that students use pencils to shade in the correct amount on the appropriate measuring device.

- Write a list of percents on the board and ask students to convert them to ratios in fraction form. Have students reduce the fractions as needed.

- Write another list of percents on the board and ask students to convert the percents to decimals.

- Stop frequently during the math skills lessons to provide students with an opportunity to practice what they have just learned. Have students work independently, with a partner, or in a small group.

- Have students form groups and distribute measuring devices and a liquid to each group. Ask students to familiarize themselves with the various measuring devices and compare the ratio and proportion of volumes that will fit, for example, in a graduated cylinder versus a beaker. Use these different-sized measuring devices and liquid volumes to also underscore the concept of percentage of error.

- Have your students get into six groups (with 2–4 students in each group) and give each group a fun-size bag of M&Ms or Skittles. Assign each group to one of the following colors: red, orange, yellow, green, blue, or brown. Ask students to count the number of candies in their assigned color in the fun-size bag. Then have students compare the size of their fun-size bag with the size of the large bag of M&Ms or Skittles. Next, ask students to set up a ratio-proportion problem to determine how many of their designated color M&Ms or Skittles must be in the large bag to have the same proportion as the fun-size bag. After they have performed the calculations, ask students to count how many of their designated color M&Ms are actually in the large bag. Ask students if their calculations were correct.

- Distribute a short quiz to assess students' understanding of the math concepts presented in this chapter.

- Use the Chapter Practice Test as a quiz or as a culminating group assignment. Invite a student from each group to write the group's solution to the problem on the board and then provide a walk-through for other groups.

Chapter 3 Developing Literacy Skills

Set Your Purpose

Upon completion of this chapter, you should ensure that students are able to meet the following learning objectives:

- Identify the elements of a complete prescription order.
- Apply calculation operations in handling prescription orders.
- Recognize the elements of a medication label.
- Apply calculation operations to information on medication labels.

Preview the Chapter

Chapter 3 provides students with an overview of the calculations that are commonly used in metric measurement conversions and dosage calculation scenarios.

- **Section 3.1: Elements of a Prescription Order**
  - focuses on identifying the various elements of a prescription
  - assists students in the recognition of elements of a hospital medication order
  - presents information on drug designation, drug labeling, days' supply, and quantity to dispense
- **Section 3.2: Prescription Directions**
  - presents the common terminology and abbreviations used in pharmacy calculations, including those used in patient directions

Plan Ahead

Prior to teaching this chapter, consider the following recommendations:

- Turn to the Handouts section and photocopy (or download and print from the Internet Resource Center) the following items for later distribution to students:
  - Chapter 3, Finding Solutions, Scenario B, #9
  - Chapter 3, Finding Solutions, Scenario B, #10
- Gather the following supplies that you will need to teach this chapter:
  - dry-erase markers for the whiteboard or chalk for the blackboard
  - markers for overhead transparencies
  - paper for practicing math problems in groups
  - a set of simple calculators (to ensure preprogrammed calculators are not used to cheat)
  - pencils and erasers
  - a minimum of three sets of colored pens or markers to use for grading in class (to avoid any student tampering during in-class grading)

- Assemble the following supplies that are needed to conduct the suggested activities listed below (enough supplies for each student or each group of students):
  - sample prescriptions
  - sample medication orders
  - drug bottles with a variety of pills, capsules, caplets
  - oral liquid drug bottles
  - parenteral drug vials
- Create a number of practice DEA numbers, both valid and invalid, that you can assign for students to have them determine the validity of the numbers.
- Create a number of practice prescriptions and medication orders that you can incorporate into the various practice problems in Chapter 3. Reading and interpreting these prescriptions and orders provide students with a context in which literacy must be developed prior to performing pharmacy calculations in the practice setting.
- If you plan to use small-group activities, consider predetermining the group participants so that each group has at least one student who is proficient in pharmacy terminology and abbreviations as well as pharmacy math.
- Take the time to work out each problem in your own handwriting, well ahead of time. Be sure to verify your calculations and answers. Consider keeping them in plastic sheet protectors in a three-ring binder so that you can easily:
  - remove the problems and have them in your hand while you are working the problem on the board
  - assist students while they are working out problems
  - use the problems as a model for other problems you want to work out on the board.
- For those problems that you plan on assigning to your students as homework, consider working out the problems using one or two alternative methods. That way, you are acknowledging the validity of using different approaches for students who arrive at their answers using alternative methods.

Establish a Context

Take time to prepare yourself for the lesson by thoroughly working out each of the problems you plan to use as instructional models. Based on your experience in earlier chapters, anticipate the types of questions that your students will ask. Do your best to plan your possible responses to the extent that is possible. To help students gain a greater understanding of the problems in this chapter, incorporate real-world examples using various medication bottles or vials as well as an assortment of prescriptions and medication orders. For example, give each student or group of students a prescription and a corresponding bottle of medication. Have the students determine the days' supply of the medication based on what the prescriber has ordered. Lastly, integrate small-group work as much as possible in your lessons. Many students benefit from working with other students. For struggling students, group work allows them to talk through the calculation steps with others and ask questions they may not feel comfortable asking in a large-group setting. For math-savvy students, group work allows them to show their approaches to the pharmacy calculation problems and to serve as peer helpers for struggling students. Be sure to have groups present their collaborative work by demonstrating their step-by-step calculations on the board and explaining their approach and process to the class.

Expand Your Lesson

The following section provides teaching tips and suggested activities that you may use to supplement your usual coursework instruction. The teaching tips suggest hints, alternative approaches, learning strategies, safety reminders, and outside resources for instructors to use. The suggested activities offer ideas for small-group and large-group discussion, related in-class activities, or homework exercises. As the course instructor, you are encouraged to modify these ideas to fit your teaching style and the needs of your students. Change them as time permits so that you address the multiple learning styles of your students.

Teaching Tips

- Remind students that the key to the body system icons that accompany the drug names in this chapter can be found on page xvi of the Preface.

- Refer students to Appendix C: Common Pharmacy Abbreviations and Acronyms if they need assistance in interpreting the meanings of abbreviations and acronyms used in the examples.

- Students have a tendency to get confused by the multi-step process of determining the validity of DEA numbers. Be prepared to work out multiple examples on the whiteboard and then assign additional problems for small-group and individual student practice.

- Be sure that students have a good understanding of the terms *gram*, *milligram*, *liter*, and *milliliter*, and their corresponding weights and measures.

- Provide students with as many "real-world" examples as possible. They will benefit from reading actual prescriptions, medication orders, drug labels, CSP labels, and vial labels and then determining days' supply and quantity to dispense from the information contained therein.

- Review with students the terms and abbreviations commonly used in the household and metric systems of measurement. Encourage your students to commit these abbreviations to memory by making flash cards with the abbreviation on one side of the card and the meaning on the opposite side of the card.

Suggested Activities

- Distribute the handouts to students prior to assigning the end-of-chapter exercises for their completion. Be sure that students use pencils to shade in the correct amount on the appropriate illustration.

- Using the sample valid and invalid DEA numbers that you created prior to class, record the numbers on the whiteboard. Place students into groups of two; then assign each pair several sets of DEA numbers to check their validity. Have each pair come to the whiteboard and work out the validity checks on the whiteboard.

- Using the sample prescriptions that you created prior to class, assign each student (or group of students) a prescription and a corresponding medication bottle. Have each student (or group of students) identify each component of the prescription and the medication label, and then determine the days' supply and quantity to dispense.

- Using the sample medication orders that you created prior to class, assign each student (or group of students) a medication order and a corresponding drug vial. Have each student (or group of students) identify each component of the medication order and the medication label, and then determine the days' supply and quantity to dispense.

Chapter 4   Applying Metric Measurements and Calculating Doses

Set Your Purpose

Upon completion of this chapter, you should ensure that students are able to meet the following learning objectives:

- Identify the basic units and prefixes of the metric system.
- Convert units within the metric system by moving the decimal point, using the ratio-proportion method, and using the dimensional analysis method.
- Calculate drug doses using the ratio-proportion and dimensional analysis methods.
- Calculate doses based on weight and body surface area.
- Calculate a pediatric dose using the patient's weight or age and the appropriate adult dose.

Preview the Chapter

Chapter 4 provides students with an overview of the calculations that are commonly used in metric measurement conversions and dosage calculation scenarios.

- **Section 4.1: Basic Metric Units**
  - focuses on identifying the various metric units of measure and their associated prefixes and abbreviations
  - provides problems to identify percentage strength and amount of various components and solutions frequently used in sterile compounding
- **Section 4.2: Conversions within the Metric System**
  - presents the approaches used when performing metric system conversions, such as moving the decimal point or implementing the ratio-proportion or dimensional analysis methods
- **Section 4.3: Problem Solving in the Pharmacy**
  - assists students with using the ratio-proportion and dimensional analysis methods to solve various pharmacy dosage calculation problems
- **Section 4.4: Customized Doses**
  - assists students with calculating doses based on body weight and body surface area
  - presents various methods used in calculating pediatric doses

Plan Ahead

Prior to teaching this chapter, consider the following recommendations:

- Turn to the Handouts section and photocopy (or download and print from the Internet Resource Center) the following items for later distribution to students:
  - Chapter 4, Chapter Practice Test, #8
  - Chapter 4, Chapter Practice Test, #10
  - Chapter 4, Chapter Practice Test, #14
  - Chapter 4, Chapter Practice Test, #15
  - Chapter 4, Chapter Practice Test, #16

- Gather the following supplies that you will need to teach this chapter:
  - dry-erase markers for the whiteboard or chalk for the blackboard
  - markers for overhead transparencies
  - paper for practicing math problems in groups
  - a set of simple calculators (to ensure preprogrammed calculators are not used to cheat)
  - pencils and erasers
  - a minimum of three sets of colored pens or markers to use for grading in class (to avoid any student tampering during in-class grading)
- Assemble the following supplies that are needed to conduct the suggested activities listed below (enough supplies for each student or each group of students):
  - nomogram and straight edge
  - oral syringes in various sizes
  - sterile parenteral syringes in various sizes
  - teaspoons, tablespoons, cup, pint, and a variety of other measuring devices
  - digital balance (or similar device for determining weight)
  - weighing boats
  - sodium chloride ($\geq$ 1 pound)
  - sugar ($\geq$ 1 pound)
  - an assortment of different medication bottles (liquids, tablets, capsules, etc.)
- Create a number of practice medication orders that you can incorporate into the various calculation problems in Chapter 4. Reading and interpreting these orders provide students with a context in which dosage calculations must be performed in the practice setting.
- If you plan to use small-group activities, consider predetermining the group participants so that each group has at least one student who is proficient in math.
- Take the time to work out each problem in your own handwriting, well ahead of time. Be sure to verify your calculations and answers. Consider keeping them in plastic sheet protectors in a three-ring binder so that you can easily:
  - remove the problems and have them in your hand while you are working the problem on the board
  - assist students while they are working out problems
  - use the problems as a model for other problems you want to work out on the board.
- For those problems that you plan on assigning to your students as homework, consider working out the problems using one or two alternative methods. That way, you are acknowledging the validity of using different approaches for students who arrive at their answers using alternative methods.

Establish a Context

Take time to prepare yourself for the lesson by thoroughly working out each of the problems you plan to use as instructional models. Based on your experience in earlier chapters, anticipate the types of questions that your students will ask. Do your best to plan your possible responses to the extent that is possible. To help students gain a greater understanding of the problems in this chapter, incorporate real-world examples using various weights and measures, as well as measuring tools. For example, give each student or group of students a nomogram and straight edge and ask them to determine a pediatric dose based on body surface area. Lastly, integrate small-group work as much as possible in your lessons. Many students benefit from working with other students. For struggling students, group work allows them to talk through the calculation steps with others and ask questions they may not feel comfortable asking in a large-group setting. For math-savvy students, group work allows them to show their approaches to the pharmacy calculation problems and to serve as peer helpers for struggling students. Be sure to have groups present their collaborative work by demonstrating their step-by-step calculations on the board and explaining their approach and process to the class.

Expand Your Lesson

The following section provides teaching tips and suggested activities that you may use to supplement your usual coursework instruction. The teaching tips suggest hints, alternative approaches, learning strategies, safety reminders, and outside resources for instructors to use. The suggested activities offer ideas for small-group and large-group discussion, related in-class activities, or homework exercises. As the course instructor, you are encouraged to modify these ideas to fit your teaching style and the needs of your students. Change them as time permits so that you address the multiple learning styles of your students.

Teaching Tips

- Remind students that the key to the body system icons that accompany the drug names in this chapter can be found on page xvi of the Preface.
- Refer students to Appendix C: Common Pharmacy Abbreviations and Acronyms if they need assistance in interpreting the meanings of abbreviations and acronyms used in the examples.
- Students have a tendency to get confused by the variety of methods for calculating pediatric doses. Be sure to review the different children's dosing methods; then conduct a class discussion about potential problems related to underdosing or overdosing due to the differences in dosing methods. Remind students that Young's Rule, Fried's Rule, and Clark's Rule are antiquated dosing methods that are no longer used due to the potential for dosing error. Reinforce to students that modern children's dosing is calculated based on either the child's body weight or body surface area (BSA).
- Be sure that students have a good understanding of the terms *gram*, *milligram*, *liter*, and *milliliter*, and their corresponding weights and measures.
- Provide students with as many "real-world" examples as possible. They will benefit from performing calculations that require them to read prescriptions, medication orders, drug labels, CSP labels, and vial labels and then determine dosage volumes from the information contained therein.
- Review with students the terms and abbreviations commonly used in the household and metric systems of measurement.
- Be sure that students have a solid understanding of common conversions including kg ↔ lb, mL ↔ tsp, mL ↔ tbsp, mL ↔ pt, mL ↔ gal, mcg ↔ mg, mg ↔ g, °F ↔ °C, etc.

Suggested Activities

- Distribute the handouts to students prior to the start of the Chapter Practice Test. Be sure that students use pencils to shade in the correct amount on the appropriate measuring device illustration.

- Gather a large variety of different pharmacy measurement instruments such as oral dosing spoons, oral syringes (1 mL , 3 mL, 5 mL, and 10 mL sizes), household measuring tools (teaspoon, tablespoon, ½ cup, cup, pint, gallon), metric volume measures (pint, liter), sterile parenteral syringes (1 mL, 3 mL, 5 mL, 10 mL, 20 mL, 60 mL). Have students perform calculations such as those found in the end-of-chapter exercises or in the Chapter 4 Practice Test. Once they have performed the calculations, have them select the most appropriate measuring device and size.

- Assign a student or group of students to calculate various doses using the strength or concentration on the prescription or medication bottle.

  Divide students into four groups, and assign each group to weigh out the following amounts into a weighing boat and set it aside.

  – Group 1: sodium chloride 227 g

  – Group 2: sodium chloride ¾ lb

  – Group 3: sugar ⅓ lb

  – Group 4: sugar 33.75 g

  Then have students weigh out the following amounts into a separate weighing boat and set it aside.

  – Group 1: sodium chloride ½ lb

  – Group 2: sodium chloride 33.75 g

  – Group 3: sugar 302.7 g

  – Group 4: sugar ¾ lb

  Finally, have students mix the amounts in their two weighing boats and answer the following questions:

  – Group 1: What is the total number of grams of sodium chloride in the weighing boat?

  – Group 2: What is the total number of pounds of sodium chloride in the weighing boat?

  – Group 3: What is the total number of grams of sugar in the weighing boat?

  – Group 4: What is the total number of pounds of sugar in the weighing boat?

- As students become more familiar with the types of calculations discussed in this chapter, consider developing their critical thinking skills by first calculating the volume of an adult dose of a parenteral medication (e.g., gentamicin 40 mg/mL; 200 mg dose); then have them determine a dose of gentamicin using the pediatric formulation (e.g., gentamicin 10 mg/mL). Ask them to determine the amount of pediatric formula gentamicin they must draw up to give a single dose of gentamicin based on the following physician order:

  Gentamicin 1.5 mg/kg IV q8h for a baby that weighs 3.5 lb

Chapter 5 Using Household Measure in Pharmacy Calculations

Set Your Purpose

Upon completion of this chapter, you should ensure that students are able to meet the following learning objectives:

- Identify units of household measure and convert between them.
- Solve medication problems by using household measure and the metric system.
- Convert body weight between kilograms and pounds.
- Determine pediatric doses using dosing tables.
- Calculate the amount of medication to be dispensed.
- Calculate temperature conversions between Celsius and Fahrenheit.

Preview the Chapter

Chapter 5 provides students with an overview of the calculations that are commonly used in household and metric measurement conversions, dosage calculations, and temperature conversions.

- **Section 5.1: Household Measure**
    - focuses on identifying the various household units of measure and their associated abbreviations
    - provides problems to convert between the household and metric systems of measurement
- **Section 5.2: Oral Doses**
    - presents the various methods for determining and measuring oral doses
- **Section 5.3: Temperature Measurement**
    - assists students with calculating temperature conversions between the Celsius and Fahrenheit systems

Plan Ahead

Prior to teaching this chapter, consider the following recommendations:

- Turn to the Handouts section and photocopy (or download and print from the Internet Resource Center) the following items for later distribution to students:
    - Chapter 5, Finding Solutions, Scenario A, #4
    - Chapter 5, Finding Solutions, Scenario B, #8
    - Chapter 5, Chapter Practice Test, #11
    - Chapter 5, Chapter Practice Test, #12
    - Chapter 5, Chapter Practice Test, #18
    - Chapter 5, Chapter Practice Test, #19
- Gather the following supplies that you will need to teach this chapter:
    - dry-erase markers for the whiteboard or chalk for the blackboard
    - markers for overhead transparencies

- paper for practicing math problems in groups
- a set of simple calculators (to ensure preprogrammed calculators are not used to cheat)
- pencils and erasers
- a minimum of three sets of colored pens or markers to use for grading in class (to avoid any student tampering during in-class grading)
- Assemble the following supplies that are needed to conduct the suggested activities listed below (enough supplies for each student or each group of students):
  - digital thermometers
  - oral syringes in various sizes
  - beakers (one for each group)
  - teaspoons, tablespoons, cup, pint, and a variety of other measuring devices
  - water for irrigation
  - temperature chart similar to what is used on page 164 of the student textbook
  - an assortment of different medication bottles (liquids, tablets, capsules, etc.)
- Create a number of prescriptions and practice medication orders that you can incorporate into the various calculation problems in Chapter 5. Reading and interpreting prescriptions and medication orders provide students with a context in which dosage calculations must be performed in the practice setting.
- If you plan to use small-group activities, consider predetermining the group participants so that each group has at least one student who is proficient in math.
- Take the time to work out each problem in your own handwriting, well ahead of time. Be sure to verify your calculations and answers. Consider keeping them in plastic sheet protectors in a three-ring binder so that you can easily:
  - remove the problems and have them in your hand while you are working the problem on the board
  - assist students while they are working out problems
  - use the problems as a model for other problems you want to work out on the board.
- For those problems that you plan on assigning to your students as homework, consider working out the problems using one or two alternative methods. That way, you are acknowledging the validity of using different approaches for students who arrive at their answers using alternative methods.

Establish a Context

Take time to prepare yourself for the lesson by thoroughly working out each of the problems you plan to use as instructional models. Based on your experience in earlier chapters, anticipate the types of questions that your students will ask. Do your best to plan your possible responses to the extent that is possible. To help students gain a greater understanding of the problems in this chapter, incorporate real-world examples using various weights and measures, and measuring instruments. For example, assign one-half of your class to start with Celsius temperatures and the other half of the class to start with Fahrenheit temperatures. Give each student or group of students a digital thermometer and have them take the temperatures of various things (e.g., the human body, tap water, ice water, etc.) and then convert the temperatures to either Celsius or Fahrenheit. Lastly, integrate small-group work as much as possible in your lessons. Many students benefit from working with other students. For struggling students, group work allows them to talk through the calculation steps with others and ask questions they may not feel comfortable asking in a large-group setting. For math-savvy students, group work allows them to show their approaches to the pharmacy calculation problems and to serve as peer helpers for struggling students. Be sure to have groups present their collaborative work by demonstrating their step-by-step calculations on the board and explaining their approach and process to the class.

Expand Your Lesson

The following section provides teaching tips and suggested activities that you may use to supplement your usual coursework instruction. The teaching tips suggest hints, alternative approaches, learning strategies, safety reminders, and outside resources for instructors to use. The suggested activities offer ideas for small-group and large-group discussion, related in-class activities, or homework exercises. As the course instructor, you are encouraged to modify these ideas to fit your teaching style and the needs of your students. Change them as time permits so that you address the multiple learning styles of your students.

Teaching Tips

- Remind students that the key to the body system icons that accompany the drug names in this chapter can be found on page xvi of the Preface.
- Refer students to Appendix C: Common Pharmacy Abbreviations and Acronyms if they need assistance in interpreting the meanings of abbreviations and acronyms used in the examples.
- Students have a tendency to get confused by temperature conversion methods. Be sure to review the methods for calculating between the Celsius and Fahrenheit measurement systems. Remind students that the United States is one of the few major countries in the world that has not adopted the Celsius scale as a standard measurement system. It is important for them to know Celsius conversions as well as all metric and household conversions. *Note:* There are a number of formulas that may be used when performing temperature conversions. Consider familiarizing yourself with all of the methods so that you can offer alternative problem-solving methods to students who struggle with the method presented in this chapter.
- Be sure that students have a good understanding of the terms *gram, milligram, liter,* and *milliliter,* and their corresponding weights and measures.
- Provide students with as many "real-world" examples as possible. They will benefit from performing calculations that require them to read prescriptions, medication orders, drug labels, compounded sterile preparation (CSP) labels, and vial labels and then determine dosage volumes from the information contained therein.
- Review with students the terms and abbreviations commonly used in the household and metric systems of measurement.
- Be sure that students have a solid understanding of common conversions including kg ↔ lb, mL ↔ tsp, mL ↔ tbsp, mL ↔ pt, mL ↔ gal, mcg ↔ mg, mg ↔ g, °F ↔ °C, etc.

Suggested Activities

- Distribute the handouts to students prior to the start of the end-of-chapter exercises and the Chapter Practice Test. Be sure that students use pencils to shade in the correct amount on the appropriate measuring device.

- Gather a large variety of different pharmacy measurement instruments such as oral dosing spoons, oral syringes (1 mL, 3 mL, 5 mL, and 10 mL sizes), household measuring tools (teaspoon, tablespoon, ½ cup, cup, pint, gallon), metric volume measures (pint, liter), sterile parenteral syringes (1 mL, 3 mL, 5 mL, 10 mL, 20 mL, 60 mL). Have students perform calculations such as those found in the end-of-chapter exercises or Chapter Practice Test. Once they have performed the calculations, have them select the most appropriate measuring tool and size.

- Assign a student or group of students to calculate various doses using the strength or concentration on the prescription or medication bottle.

- Divide students into four groups, and assign each group to measure out the following amounts of water using the designated measuring instrument and put the amounts into a beaker:

  - Group 1: 15 mL (oral syringe)
  - Group 2: 10 mL (oral syringe)
  - Group 3: one teaspoon
  - Group 4: one tablespoon

  Then have the students measure the following amounts into the same beaker:

  - Group 1: two teaspoons
  - Group 2: one tablespoon
  - Group 3: 20 mL (oral syringe)
  - Group 4: 10 mL (oral syringe)

  Finally, have students mix the amounts into a beaker and perform calculations to answer the following questions:

  - What is the total number of milliliters in each beaker?
  - How many milliliters must you add to the beaker to have 1 oz of water?

- As students become more familiar with the types of calculations discussed in this chapter, consider developing their critical thinking skills by asking them to determine the Fahrenheit temperature of a refrigerator in your pharmacy lab. Then have them convert the temperature to the Celsius scale and record the temperature on a temperature chart. If your students do not have access to a refrigerator, ask them to determine the temperature of the room.

Chapter 6   Preparing Injectable Medications

Set Your Purpose

Upon completion of this chapter, you should ensure that students are able to meet the following learning objectives:

- Calculate the volume to be measured when given a specific dose.
- Calculate the amount of drug in a given volume.

- Identify drugs that use units as a dose designation.
- Calculate the volume of a substance that has an electrolyte as its primary ingredient.
- Determine the quantity of units in a given concentration and dose.
- Calculate the volume of insulin to be administered.

Preview the Chapter

Chapter 6 provides students with an overview of the calculations that are commonly used when preparing injectable medications in sterile compounding situations.

- **Section 6.1: Parenteral Injections and Infusions**
  - focuses on identifying the various units of measure for injectable solutions, and their associated prefixes and abbreviations
  - provides problems to instruct students in basic dosage calculation and the ratio-proportion problems that are commonly encountered when preparing parenteral medications
- **Section 6.2: Other Units of Measure**
  - presents the various methods to solve problems with calculations involving milliequivalents and units
- **Section 6.3: Solutions Using Powders**
  - assists students with calculating parenteral medications that are comprised of solution and powder components

Plan Ahead

Prior to teaching this chapter, consider the following recommendations:

- Turn to the Handouts section and photocopy (or download and print from the Internet Resource Center) the following items for later distribution to students:
  - Chapter 6, 6.1 Problem Set, #1
  - Chapter 6, 6.1 Problem Set, #2
  - Chapter 6, 6.1 Problem Set, #3
  - Chapter 6, 6.1 Problem Set, #4
  - Chapter 6, 6.1 Problem Set, #5
  - Chapter 6, 6.1 Problem Set, #6
  - Chapter 6, 6.1 Problem Set, #7
  - Chapter 6, 6.1 Problem Set, #8
  - Chapter 6, 6.1 Problem Set, #9
  - Chapter 6, 6.1 Problem Set, #10
  - Chapter 6, 6.2 Problem Set, #1
  - Chapter 6, 6.2 Problem Set, #2
  - Chapter 6, 6.2 Problem Set, #4
  - Chapter 6, 6.2 Problem Set, #6
  - Chapter 6, 6.2 Problem Set, #7
  - Chapter 6, 6.2 Problem Set, #8
  - Chapter 6, 6.2 Problem Set, #13
  - Chapter 6, 6.2 Problem Set, #14

- Chapter 6, 6.2 Problem Set, #16
- Chapter 6, Finding Solutions, Scenario A, #2
- Chapter 6, Finding Solutions, Scenario B, #6 and #7
- Chapter 6, Chapter Practice Test, #1
- Chapter 6, Chapter Practice Test, #2
- Chapter 6, Chapter Practice Test, #3
- Chapter 6, Chapter Practice Test, #4

- Gather the following supplies that you will need to teach this chapter:
  - dry-erase markers for the whiteboard or chalk for the blackboard
  - markers for overhead transparencies
  - paper for practicing math problems in groups
  - a set of simple calculators (to ensure preprogrammed calculators are not used to cheat)
  - pencils and erasers
  - a minimum of three sets of colored pens or markers to use for grading in class (to avoid any student tampering during in-class grading)

- Assemble the following supplies that are needed to conduct the suggested activities listed below (enough supplies for each student or each group of students):
  - an assortment of parenteral medication vials
  - an assortment of parenteral electrolyte vials
  - an assortment of insulin vials
  - sterile syringes in various sizes (1 mL, 3 mL, 5 mL, 10 mL, 20 mL, 30 mL, and 60 mL)
  - an assortment of parenteral vials in powdered form
  - vials of sterile water for diluent use
  - an assortment of intravenous (IV) and intravenous piggyback (IVPB) solutions and volumes

- Create a number of prescriptions and practice medication orders that you can incorporate into the various calculation problems in Chapter 6. Reading and interpreting prescriptions and medication orders provide students with a context in which dosage calculations must be performed in the practice setting.

- If you plan to use small-group activities, consider predetermining the group participants so that each group has at least one student who is proficient in math.

- Take the time to work out each problem in your own handwriting, well ahead of time. Be sure to verify your calculations and answers. Consider keeping them in plastic sheet protectors in a three-ring binder so that you can easily:
  - remove the problems and have them in your hand while you are working the problem on the board
  - assist students while they are working out problems
  - use the problems as a model for other problems you want to work out on the board.

- For those problems that you plan on assigning to your students as homework, consider working out the problems using one or two alternative methods. That way, you are acknowledging the validity of using different approaches for students who arrive at their answers using alternative methods.

Establish a Context

Take time to prepare yourself for the lesson by thoroughly working out each of the problems you plan to use as instructional models. Based on your experience in earlier chapters, anticipate the types of questions that your students will ask. Do your best to plan your possible responses to the extent that is possible. To help students gain a greater understanding of the problems in this chapter, incorporate real-world examples using various medication orders and compounded sterile preparation (CSP) labels. For example, provide students with a medication order and CSP label. Have student gather the medications and IV base solutions listed on both, and then perform the necessary calculations to determine the volume of each ingredient listed. Then have them retrieve the appropriate syringe size and draw up the correct amount of each ingredient. Lastly, integrate small-group work as much as possible in your lessons. Many students benefit from working with other students. For struggling students, group work allows them to talk through the calculation steps with others and ask questions they may not feel comfortable asking in a large-group setting. For math-savvy students, group work allows them to show their approaches to the pharmacy calculation problems and to serve as peer helpers for struggling students. Be sure to have groups present their collaborative work by demonstrating their step-by-step calculations on the board and explaining their approach and process to the class.

Expand Your Lesson

The following section provides teaching tips and suggested activities that you may use to supplement your usual coursework instruction. The teaching tips suggest hints, alternative approaches, learning strategies, safety reminders, and outside resources for instructors to use. The suggested activities offer ideas for small-group and large-group discussion, related in-class activities, or homework exercises. As the course instructor, you are encouraged to modify these ideas to fit your teaching style and the needs of your students. Change them as time permits so that you address the multiple learning styles of your students.

Teaching Tips

- Remind students that the key to the body system icons that accompany the drug names in this chapter can be found on page xvi of the Preface.
- Refer students to Appendix C: Common Pharmacy Abbreviations and Acronyms if they need assistance in interpreting the meanings of abbreviations and acronyms used in the examples.
- Students have a tendency to get confused by the various methods that are used in dosage calculation. Most pharmacy calculations can be solved by using simple dosage calculations (e.g., addition or division problems), the ratio-proportion method, or the dimensional analysis method. Students have a tendency to develop a natural preference for one method. Although it is important for students to have a basic understanding of all of the methods used in pharmacy calculations, some students will struggle with one or more of these problem-solving methods. Once students find their preferred method of problem solving, allowing them to use that method of problem solving may avoid a great deal of confusion and frustration for students.
- Be sure that students have a good understanding of the terms *gram*, *milligram*, *milliequivalent*, *unit*, *liter*, and *milliliter*, and their corresponding weights and measures.

- Provide students with as many "real-world" examples as possible. They will benefit from performing calculations that require them to read prescriptions, medication orders, drug labels, CSP labels, and vial labels and then to determine dosage volumes from the information contained therein.
- Review with students the terms and abbreviations commonly used in the household and metric systems of measurement.
- Be sure that students have a solid understanding of common conversions including kg ↔ lb, mL ↔ tsp, mcg ↔ mg, and mg ↔ g.

Suggested Activities

- Distribute the handouts to students prior to the start of the problem sets, end-of-chapter exercises, and Chapter Practice Test. Be sure that students use pencils to shade in the correct amount on the appropriate measuring device.
- Gather a large variety of sterile syringes: 1 mL , 3 mL, 5 mL, 10 mL, 20 mL, 30 mL, and 60 mL sizes. Have students perform calculations such as those found in the end-of-chapter exercises or Chapter Practice Test. Once they have performed the calculations, have them select the most appropriate syringe size.
- Assign a student or group of students to calculate various doses using the strength or concentration on the vial.
- Divide students into four groups, and assign each group to draw up the following amount of sterile water for injection:
  - Group 1: 4.8 mL
  - Group 2: 5 mL
  - Group 3: 9.7 mL
  - Group 4: 10 mL

  Give the students the following medication vials:
  - Group 1: ampicillin 500 mg
  - Group 2: ampicillin 500 mg
  - Group 3: ampicillin 1 g
  - Group 4: ampicillin 1 g

  Then have students inject the sterile water diluent into their assigned vials and answer the following questions:

  - What is the suggested diluent amount for your vial? (This can be found on the ampicillin vial label.)

  - What is the actual total volume in the vial once you added the diluent?

  - How much of that volume was comprised of powder?

  - What is the actual concentration of the reconstituted vial?

- As students become more familiar with the types of calculations discussed in this chapter, consider developing their critical thinking skills by asking them to first read the medication order and then prepare a CSP label for the medication. Once these tasks have been completed, have students gather the necessary medication and base solutions and draw up the correct volumes to prepare the CSP.

Chapter 7   Preparing Parenteral Solutions

Set Your Purpose

Upon completion of this chapter, you should ensure that students are able to meet the following learning objectives:

- Calculate the amount of medication in a solution based on a given percentage strength.
- Calculate the percentage strength of medication in a given solution.
- Describe the types of IV sets by drop factor.
- Calculate IV drip rates and flow rates using various IV sets.
- Estimate and calculate time for IV administration.
- Calculate rates of IV infusion and IV piggyback infusion.

Preview the Chapter

Chapter 7 provides students with an overview of the calculations that are commonly used in sterile compounding situations.

- **Section 7.1: Percentage and Ratio Strength Dilutions**
  - focuses on the types of calculations that are used to compare different strengths of compounds
  - provides problems to identify percentage strength and amount of various components and solutions frequently used in sterile compounding
- **Section 7.2: IV Flow Rates**
  - presents the essential calculations used by sterile compounding personnel to solve problems related to dosage, amount administered, and days' supply of compounded sterile preparations
- **Section 7.3: Drop Factor and Infusion Rates**
  - assists students with performing calculations based on the prescribed IV tubing's drop factor

Plan Ahead

Prior to teaching this chapter, consider the following recommendations:

- Turn to the Handouts section and photocopy (or download and print from the Internet Resource Center) the following items for later distribution to students:
  - Chapter 7, Chapter Practice Test, #23
  - Chapter 7, Chapter Practice Test, #24
  - Chapter 7, Chapter Practice Test, #25
  - Chapter 7, Chapter Practice Test, #26
  - Chapter 7, Chapter Practice Test, #27
  - Chapter 7, Chapter Practice Test, #28
  - Chapter 7, Chapter Practice Test, #29
  - Chapter 7, Chapter Practice Test, #30

- Gather the following supplies that you will need to teach this chapter:
  - dry-erase markers for the whiteboard or chalk for the blackboard
  - markers for overhead transparencies
  - paper for practicing math problems in groups
  - a set of simple calculators (to ensure preprogrammed calculators are not used to cheat)
  - pencils and erasers
  - a minimum of three sets of colored pens or markers to use for grading in class (to avoid any student tampering during in-class grading)
- Assemble the following supplies that are needed to conduct the suggested activities listed below:
  - 5 g of sugar in a weighing boat
  - 100 mL of water in a beaker
  - D_5W IV solution bags in the following volumes: 50 mL, 100 mL, 500 mL, and 1000 mL
  - IV sets with the following drop factors: 10 gtts/mL, 20 gtts/mL, and 60 gtts/mL
  - 500 mL (or larger) solution of any types
  - 250 mL (or larger) beaker
  - normal saline solution in the following volumes: 50 mL, 100 mL, 250 mL, 300 mL, 500 mL, 1000 mL, and 1250 mL
- Create a number of practice medication orders that you can incorporate into the various calculation problems in Chapter 7. Reading and interpreting these orders provide students with a context in which dosage calculations must be performed in the practice setting.
- Obtain IV set tubing in several drop factors (10 gtts/mL, 20 gtts/mL, 60 gtts/mL) for an in-class demonstration and a IV solution bag (any type).
- If you plan to use small-group activities, consider predetermining the group participants so that each group has at least one student who is proficient in math.
- Take the time to work out each problem in your own handwriting, well ahead of time. Be sure to verify your calculations and answers. Consider keeping them in plastic sheet protectors in a three-ring binder so that you can easily:
  - remove the problems and have them in your hand while you are working the problem on the board
  - assist students while they are working out problems
  - use the problems as a model for other problems you want to work out on the board.
- For those problems that you plan on assigning to your students as homework, consider working out the problems using one or two alternative methods. That way, you are acknowledging the validity of using different approaches for students who arrive at their answers using alternative methods.

Establish a Context

Take time to prepare yourself for the lesson by thoroughly working out each of the problems you plan to use as instructional models. Based on your experience in earlier chapters, anticipate the types of questions that your students will ask. Do your best to plan your possible responses to the extent that is possible. To help students gain a greater understanding of the problems in this chapter, incorporate real-world examples using various weights and measures, or actual stock IV solutions. For example, give each student or group of students an IV or IVPB solution and ask them to calculate the number of grams or milliliters for each component of the solution. Lastly, integrate small-group work as much as possible in your lessons. Many students benefit from working with other students. For struggling students, group work allows them to talk through the calculation steps with others and ask questions they may not feel comfortable asking in a large-group setting. For math-savvy students, group work allows them to show their approaches to the pharmacy calculation problems and to serve as peer helpers for struggling students. Be sure to have groups present their collaborative work by demonstrating their step-by-step calculations on the board and explaining their approach and process to the class.

Expand Your Lesson

The following section provides teaching tips and suggested activities that you may use to supplement your usual coursework instruction. The teaching tips suggest hints, alternative approaches, learning strategies, safety reminders, and outside resources for instructors to use. The suggested activities offer ideas for small-group and large-group discussion, related in-class activities, or homework exercises. As the course instructor, you are encouraged to modify these ideas to fit your teaching style and the needs of your students. Change them as time permits so that you address the multiple learning styles of your students.

Teaching Tips

- Remind students that the key to the body system icons that accompany the drug names in this chapter can be found on page xvi of the Preface.
- Refer students to Appendix C: Common Pharmacy Abbreviations and Acronyms if they need assistance in interpreting the meanings of abbreviations and acronyms used in the examples.
- Be sure that students have a good understanding of the terms *gram*, *milligram*, *liter*, and *milliliter*, and their corresponding weights and measures.
- Provide students with as many "real-world" examples as possible. They will benefit from performing calculations that require them to read CSP and vial labels and then determine dosage volumes from the information contained therein.
- Be sure that students know common IV base solutions and their abbreviations, such as dextrose 5% in water (D_5W), 0.9% sodium chloride (normal saline or NS), and lactated Ringer's (LR) solution.
- Review with students the terms and abbreviations of base components and additives commonly used to create TPN: sterile water (SW), dextrose (D), Aminosyn (AA), Liposyn, sodium (Na), potassium (K), phosphate (PO_4), magnesium (Mg), and calcium (Ca).

Suggested Activities

- Distribute the handouts to students prior to the start of the Chapter Practice Test. Be sure that students use pencils to shade in the correct amount on the appropriate syringe illustration.

- Show students the 5 g of premeasured sugar in the weighing boat and the 100 mL of premeasured water in a beaker. Then ask students to visualize 5 g of sugar in 100 mL of fluid as the equivalent of D_5W (i.e., 5 g of dextrose/100 mL).

- After reviewing the calculations in Section 7.1, display the 50 mL, 100 mL, 500 mL, and 1000 mL bags of D_5W IV solution. Then ask students to perform the necessary calculations to determine how many grams of sugar are in each of the IV bags displayed.

- Prepare a demonstration on drop size using the different drop sets, the 500 mL (or larger) bag of solution, and the 250 mL (or larger) beaker. Begin by having students gather around a table holding the supplies. Then spike the bag with the 10 gtts/mL tubing. Next, manipulate the tubing's roll clamp to slowly release fluid from the tip of the tubing, allowing it to fall (drop by drop) into the beaker. Repeat the demonstration with the other IV sets so the students can visualize the different drop sizes delivered by each set.

- Divide students into pairs or trios, and assign each group one of the following volumes of normal saline: 50 mL, 100 mL, 250 mL, 300 mL, 500 mL, 1000 mL, or 1250 mL. Be sure to remind students that normal saline is equivalent to 0.9% sodium chloride, or 0.9 g/100 mL. Then ask each group to perform calculations to determine the number of grams of sodium chloride contained in the assigned volume of normal saline. Have each group weigh out the appropriate amount of sodium chloride in a weighing boat.

- Using the different drop factor tubing, demonstrate drop size delivered by each tubing by spiking an IV bag with the tubing and slowly dripping fluid from the tubing onto a one-inch stack of gauze or paper towel.

- As students become more familiar with the types of calculations discussed in this chapter, consider developing their critical thinking skills by determining the actual concentration of various w/v solutions. Prior to posing the problem, inform students that if they were to weigh enough sugar to make a solution of 100 mL of $D_{10}W$ (i.e., 10 g), a significant amount of fluid would be displaced by adding the sugar to 100 mL of water. Proceed to then ask students to determine the actual concentration of the solution if they poured 10 g of sugar into 100 mL of water. Ask students to calculate the actual volume of water they should put into the beaker in order to mix with 10 g of sugar to have a final solution with a total volume of 100 mL and a concentration of $D_{10}W$.

Chapter 8   Using Special Calculations in Compounding

Set Your Purpose

Upon completion of this chapter, you should ensure that students are able to meet the following learning objectives:

- Calculate the amount of each ingredient needed to enlarge a formula or recipe.
- Calculate the amount of each ingredient needed to reduce a formula or recipe.
- Compute the amount of two strengths of active ingredient needed to prepare a product whose concentration lies between the two extremes.

- Determine the amount of two ingredients using the weight-in-weight formula.
- Determine the amount of concentrate and diluent needed to prepare a special dilution.

Preview the Chapter

Chapter 8 provides students with an overview of the various calculations that are used in pharmacy compounding situations.

- **Section 8.1: Compound Formulas**
    - focuses on the types of calculations that are used to reduce or enlarge formulas of existing recipes
- **Section 8.2: Alligations**
    - presents calculations that are occasionally used by pharmacy technicians who may be required to mix two different strengths of the same active ingredient of a drug or solution in order to make a desired strength
- **Section 8.3: Weight-in-Weight (w/w) Calculations**
    - assists students with performing calculations that may be required when compounding two or more active ingredients in which the ingredients are in solid form
- **Section 8.4: Special Dilutions**
    - introduces students to the calculations used to prepare compounded preparations when commercial preparations are not readily available

Plan Ahead

Prior to teaching this chapter, consider the following recommendations:

- Turn to the Handouts section and photocopy (or download and print from the Internet Resource Center) the following items for later distribution to students:
    - Chapter 8, Chapter Practice Test, #1b
    - Chapter 8, Chapter Practice Test, #1c
    - Chapter 8, Chapter Practice Test, #2b
    - Chapter 8, Chapter Practice Test, #2c
    - Chapter 8, Chapter Practice Test, #3b
    - Chapter 8, Chapter Practice Test, #3c
    - Chapter 8, Practice Test, #5
- Gather the following supplies that you will need to teach this chapter:
    - dry-erase markers for the whiteboard or chalk for the blackboard
    - markers for overhead transparencies
    - paper for practicing math problems in groups
    - a set of simple calculators (to ensure preprogrammed calculators are not used to cheat)
    - pencils and erasers
    - a minimum of three sets of colored pens or markers to use for grading in class (to avoid any student tampering during in-class grading)
- If you plan to use small-group activities, consider predetermining the group participants so that each group has at least one student who is proficient in math.

- Take the time to work out each problem in your own handwriting, well ahead of time. Be sure to verify your calculations and answers. Consider keeping them in plastic sheet protectors in a three-ring binder so that you can easily:
  - remove the problems and have them in your hand while you are working the problem on the board
  - assist students while they are working out problems
  - use the problems as a model for other problems you want to work out on the board.
- For those problems that you plan on assigning to your students as homework, consider working out the problems using one or two alternative methods. That way, you are acknowledging the validity of using different approaches for students who arrive at their answers using alternative methods.
- Determine which, if any, lab activities you will do that will support your students in application of the pharmacy calculations presented in Chapter 8. Gather the necessary supplies for those activities. For instance, the ingredients necessary to prepare cookies from scratch (e.g., flour, sugar, butter, eggs, measuring cups, measuring spoons, mixing bowl, etc.); the ingredients necessary to prepare a pharmacy compound (e.g., appropriate amounts of zinc oxide, calamine, hydrocortisone, and talc powders), a 50 g weighing boat and a digital scale for each group; enough IV bags so that each group has a bag of D_5W and $D_{70}W$; or enough of the various syringe sizes necessary for each student to simulate the volumes that correspond to the additive volumes determined in the TPN calculation.
- Using the TPN forms in the student textbook as a template, create sample TPN forms for your students by changing the amounts of dextrose, Aminosyn, Liposyn, and additives.

Establish a Context

Take time to prepare yourself for the lesson by thoroughly working out each of the problems you plan to use as instructional models. Based on your experience in earlier chapters, anticipate the types of questions that your students will ask. Do your best to plan your possible responses to the extent that is possible. To help students gain a greater understanding of the problems in this chapter, incorporate real-world examples using various weights and measures, or actual stock IV solutions. For example, give each student or group of students a stock solution of D_5W and a stock solution of $D_{70}W$; ask them to calculate the number of milliliters of each stock solution that would be needed to prepare 500 mL of a $D_{13}W$ solution. Some students find Section 8.2: Alligations particularly confusing. With that in mind, be sure to allow additional time in your course planning to allow for the questions and extra practice that accompany challenging content. Lastly, integrate small-group work as much as possible in your lessons. Many students benefit from working with other students. For struggling students, group work allows them to talk through the calculation steps with others and ask questions they may not feel comfortable asking in a large-group setting. For math-savvy students, group work allows them to show their approaches to the pharmacy calculation problems and to serve as peer helpers for struggling students. Be sure to have groups present their collaborative work by demonstrating their step-by-step calculations on the board and explaining their approach and process to the class.

Expand Your Lesson

The following section provides teaching tips and suggested activities that you may use to supplement your usual coursework instruction. The teaching tips suggest hints, alternative approaches, learning strategies, safety reminders, and outside resources for instructors to use. The suggested activities offer ideas for small-group and large-group discussion, related in-class activities, or homework exercises. As the course instructor, you are encouraged to modify these ideas to fit your teaching style and the needs of your students. Change them as time permits so that you address the multiple learning styles of your students.

Teaching Tips

- Remind students that the key to the body system icons that accompany the drug names in this chapter can be found on page xvi of the Preface.

- Refer students to Appendix C: Common Pharmacy Abbreviations and Acronyms if they need assistance in interpreting the meanings of abbreviations and acronyms used in the examples.

- Be sure that students have a good understanding of the terms *gram*, *milligram*, *liter*, and *milliliter*, and their corresponding weights and measures.

- Due to the multi-step, complex calculation process, alligation problems tend to be particularly confusing for students. It is advisable to work several examples of alligation problems on the board for students prior to assigning this type of problem for self-study.

- For alligation problems, encourage students to check their work by performing the optional step of adding together the volume of both strengths of dextrose and the volume of sterile water. If the three volumes do not add up to equal the desired total volume, they have made an error and must rework their calculations.

- Due to the multi-step, complex calculation process, TPN problems tend to be particularly confusing for students. It is advisable to work several examples of TPN problems on the board, or on preprinted handouts, for the students prior to assigning this type of problem for self-study.

Suggested Activities

- Distribute the handouts to students prior to the start of the Chapter Practice Test. Be sure that students use pencils to shade in the correct amount on the appropriate syringe.

- Have students weigh and measure the ingredients needed to bake a batch of cookies. Have some students perform calculations necessary to reduce the formula in order to prepare a partial batch, while other students perform the calculations necessary to prepare a double batch of cookies. Have students weigh and measure the reduced-formula or enlarged-formula ingredients that they have determined from their calculations.

- Break the students into three groups. For each group, distribute one of the following substances: zinc oxide powder 5 g, calamine powder 5 g, or hydrocortisone 0.5 g. Ask each group to weigh out their assigned ingredient on a weighing boat and temporarily set the measured amount aside. Tell the groups that a single compound will be made from each group's assigned ingredient, plus the addition of talc. To prepare this compound, each group will combine their weighed ingredients into a single, large weighing boat and then add the talc QSAD to 50 g total. Instruct the groups to calculate how many grams of talc will be needed to create the compound. The first group that completes this calculation should weigh the necessary amount of talc in a weighing boat. Once all groups have completed their calculations, combine all ingredients into a single weighing boat. Then ask each group to determine the percent strength of the zinc oxide, calamine, and hydrocortisone components for the final 50 g compound.

- Divide the class into groups of three or four students. Give each group the following stock IV solutions: one D_5W 500 mL bag and one $D_{70}W$ 500 mL bag. After reviewing the calculations in Section 8.2: Alligations, ask students to read the labeling on the IV bags, and then perform the necessary calculations to determine how much of each solution (in grams and in milliliters) they will need in order to prepare the following final solutions: D_7W 150 mL, $D_{12}W$ 250 mL, $D_{14}W$ 250 mL.

- Distribute the sample TPN orders and have students perform all of the calculations. Ask students to draw back the plunger on empty syringes to reflect the volume of each additive that is to be drawn up for the TPN.

Chapter 9   Using Business Math in the Pharmacy

Set Your Purpose

Upon completion of this chapter, you should ensure that students are able to meet the following learning objectives:

- Describe overhead and calculate overhead cost.
- Understand the distinction between net profit and gross profit.
- Calculate markup and the markup rate.
- Compute discounts.
- Apply average wholesale price to profit calculations.
- Calculate inventory turnover.
- Determine depreciation.

Preview the Chapter

Chapter 9 provides students with a broad overview of the business-related calculations commonly used in a retail pharmacy setting. The chapter is broken down into three sections:

- **Section 9.1: Calculations Related to Business**
  - focuses on the types of calculations used to determine gross, net, and desired profit, as well as selling prices and discounts

- **Section 9.2: Insurance Reimbursements for Prescriptions**
  - presents detailed calculations used by pharmacy personnel to solve problems related to average wholesale price (AWP), capitation fees, and profit margin

- **Section 9.3: Pharmacy Inventory**
  - discusses the procedures for managing inventory, including such topics as days' supply, turnover rate, and reorder amounts

Plan Ahead

Prior to teaching this chapter, consider the following recommendations:

- Turn to the Handouts section and photocopy (or download and print from the Internet Resource Center) the following items for later distribution to students:
  - Chapter 9, Finding Solutions, Scenario A
  - Chapter 9, Finding Solutions, Scenario B
- Gather the following supplies that you will need to teach this chapter:
  - dry-erase markers for the whiteboard or chalk for the blackboard
  - markers for overhead transparencies
  - paper for practicing math problems in groups
  - a set of simple calculators (to ensure preprogrammed calculators are not used to cheat)
  - pencils and erasers
  - a minimum of three sets of colored pens or markers to use for grading in class (to avoid any student tampering during in-class grading)
- If you plan to use small-group activities, consider predetermining the group participants so that each group has at least one student who is proficient in math.
- Take the time to work out each problem in your own handwriting, well ahead of time. Be sure to verify your calculations and answers. Consider keeping them in plastic sheet protectors in a three-ring binder so that you can easily:
  - remove the problems and have them in your hand while you are working the problem on the board
  - assist students while they are working out problems
  - use the problems as a model for other problems you want to work out on the board.
- For those problems that you plan on assigning to your students as homework, consider working out the problems using one or two alternative methods. That way, you are acknowledging the validity of using different approaches for students who arrive at their answers using alternative methods.
- Determine which, if any, lab activities you will do that will support your students in application of the pharmacy calculations presented in Chapter 9. Gather the necessary supplies for those activities—for example, play money, OTC items, etc.
- Procure a cash register for use in your pharmacy lab. Check with local pharmacies and supermarkets to determine if these facilities would be willing to donate a used cash register to your program. You can also find reasonably priced cash registers from any office supply store.
- Create price stickers for use in your pharmacy lab. Price stickers are available from Internet sources such as Total Pharmacy Supply, MediDose, and Integral Solutions. You can also make custom price stickers using any computer-based labeling program available from an office supply store.
- Obtain play money from any office supply store or online from The Activity Village website.

- Ask local pharmacies to collect empty pharmacy drug bottles and other supplies and donate them to your program. Fill the drug bottles with beans or candy to simulate pills and tablets. Place price stickers on the bottles to simulate pharmacy practice scenarios.
- Use the inventory order forms on pages 301–303 of the student textbook as a template to create your own inventory tables for students to practice their skills.

Establish a Context

Take time to prepare yourself for the lesson by thoroughly working out each of the problems you plan to use as instructional models. Based on your experience in earlier chapters, anticipate the types of questions that your students will ask. Do your best to plan your possible responses to the extent that is possible. To help students gain a greater understanding of the problems in this chapter, incorporate real-world examples using play money, or actual stock pharmacy items. In addition, integrate small-group work as much as possible in your lessons. Many students benefit from working with other students. For struggling students, group work allows them to talk through the calculation steps with others and ask questions they may not feel comfortable asking in a large-group setting. For math-savvy students, group work allows them to show their approaches to the pharmacy calculation problems and to serve as peer helpers for struggling students. Be sure to have groups present their collaborative work by demonstrating their step-by-step calculations on the board and explaining their approach and process to the class.

Expand Your Lesson

The following section provides teaching tips and suggested activities that you may use to supplement your usual coursework instruction. The teaching tips suggest hints, alternative approaches, learning strategies, safety reminders, and outside resources for instructors to use. The suggested activities offer ideas for small-group and large-group discussion, related in-class activities, or homework exercises. As the course instructor, you are encouraged to modify these ideas to fit your teaching style and the needs of your students. Change them as time permits so that you address the multiple learning styles of your students.

Teaching Tips

- Remind students that the key to the body system icons that accompany the drug names in this chapter can be found on page xvi of the Preface.
- Be sure that students have a good understanding of the terms *pharmacy benefits manager, average wholesale price, dispensing fee,* and *capitation fee.* Students should also know how these terms apply to retail pharmacy practice.
- Re-create real-world scenarios in your classroom that incorporate the pharmacy calculations presented in Chapter 9. With that in mind, be sure to give students the opportunity to determine discount prices, practice using the cash register to ring up sales, and serve "customers."
- Devote some classroom discussion to the concept of product markup. Students are often surprised by the fact that some pharmacy items are marked up well over 100% whereas other items have hardly any markup at all. Explain to students that various factors influence item markup, including price contracts with wholesalers, insurance reimbursement amounts, and supply and demand issues.

- Spend time discussing the concept of depreciation, a topic that is challenging for some students. Again, it is useful to put this concept into a real-world context—for example, the depreciation of a car or a computer. Explain to students that the moment they purchase either a car or a computer the value of the item drops. This concept also applies to the pharmacy setting in which the value of pharmacy equipment, furniture, etc. also drops or depreciates over time.

Suggested Activities

- Distribute the handouts to students prior to the assignment of the Finding Solutions section.
- Give each student or group of students a box of pharmacy stock items marked with price stickers (e.g., OTC products such as aspirin, milk of magnesia, toothpaste, etc.). Tell students that your pharmacy is going to have a 25%-off sale, and ask them to calculate new prices for each item in preparation for the sale.
- Using the cash register and play money that you procured, assign one student to serve as pharmacy cashier and ask the other students to "purchase" several items from the cashier. Once all of the students have completed their sales transactions, have students determine the total sales for the day.
- Assign a group of students to a particular section of the pharmacy lab. Ask them to perform an inventory count and determine the actual inventory amount (in dollars) that is on the shelves in their assigned section. Then ask the students to record their totals on the board and tally up the total amount of inventory on the pharmacy lab's shelves.
- Assign a group of students to a particular section of the pharmacy lab. Ask them to use the inventory order forms to determine the reorder amounts for the drugs and pharmacy stock in their sections.

Handouts

Chapter 1

Chapter 2

Chapter 3

Chapter 4

Chapter 5

Chapter 6

Chapter 7

Chapter 8

Chapter 9

Answer Keys for Handouts   **127**

Finding Solutions, Scenario D, #9

Directions: Fill in the correct volume to be administered on the measuring device.

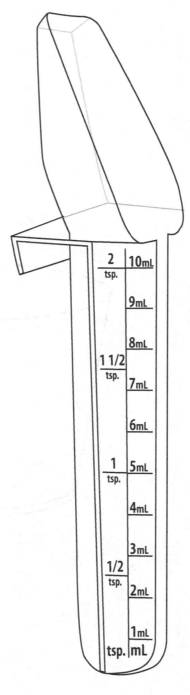

Dosing Spoon

Finding Solutions, Scenario A, #1

Directions: Select the measuring device that will be used and fill in the volume to be administered with each dose.

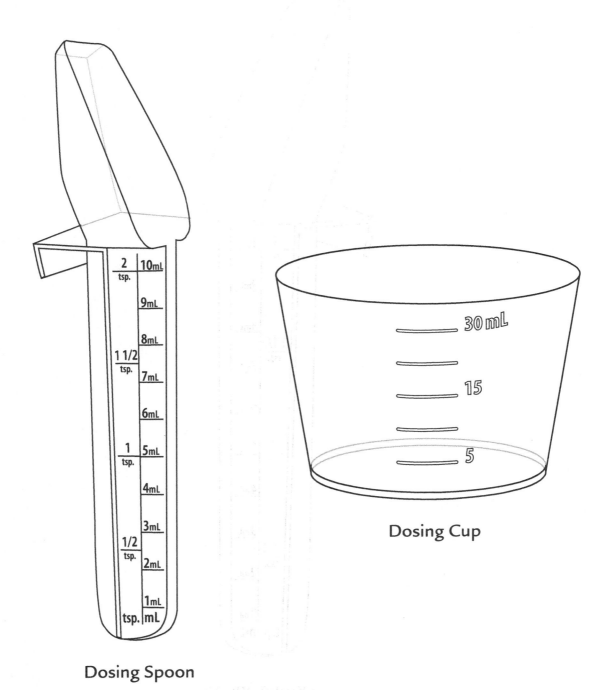

Dosing Spoon

Dosing Cup

Finding Solutions, Scenario B, #9

Directions: Select the measuring device that will be used and fill in the volume to be administered with each dose.

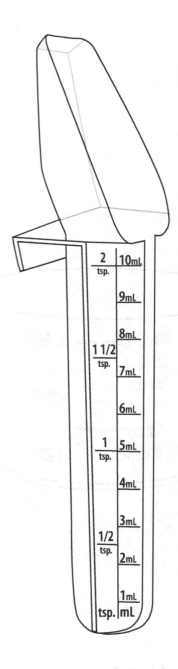

Dosing Spoon

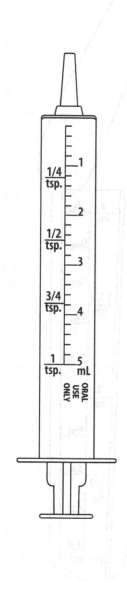

Oral Syringe

Finding Solutions, Scenario B, #10

Directions: Select the measuring device that will be used and fill in the volume to be administered with each dose.

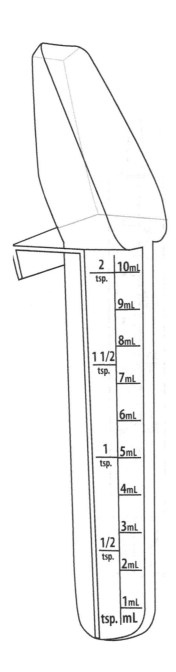

2 tsp.	10mL
	9mL
	8mL
1 1/2 tsp.	7mL
	6mL
1 tsp.	5mL
	4mL
	3mL
1/2 tsp.	2mL
	1mL
tsp.	mL

Dosing Spoon

30 cc ———— 2 TBSP
25 cc ————
20 cc ————
15 cc ———— 1 TBSP
10 cc ————
5 cc ———— 1 TSP

Medicine Cup

Chapter Practice Test, #8

Directions: Select the measuring device that will be used and fill in the volume to be administered with each dose.

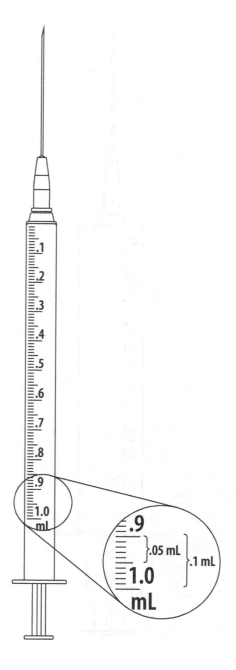

1 mL Syringe

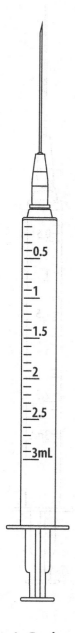

3 mL Syringe

Chapter Practice Test, #10

Directions: Select the measuring device that will be used and fill in the volume to be administered with each dose.

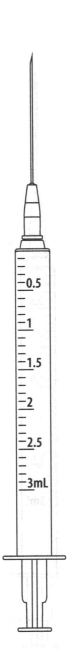

3 mL Syringe

10 mL Syringe

Chapter Practice Test, #14

Directions: Select the measuring device that will be used and fill in the volume to be administered with each dose.

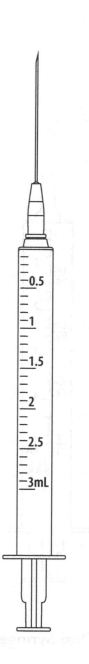

3 mL Syringe

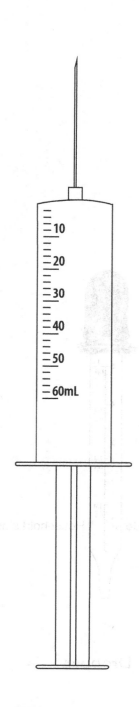

60 mL Syringe

Chapter Practice Test, #15

Directions: Select the measuring device that will be used and fill in the volume to be administered with each dose.

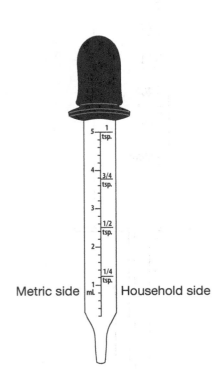

Metric side Household side

Dropper

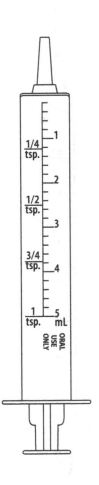

Oral Syringe

Chapter Practice Test, #16

Directions: Select the measuring device that will be used and fill in the volume to be administered with each dose.

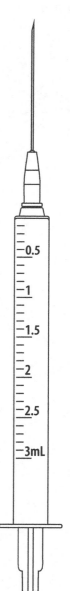

0.5

1

1.5

2

2.5

3mL

1

2

3

4

5

6

7

8

9

10mL

3 mL Syringe   10 mL Syringe

Finding Solutions, Scenario A, #4

Directions: Fill in the correct volume to be administered on the measuring device.

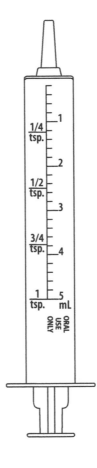

5 mL Oral Syringe

Finding Solutions, Scenario B, #8

Directions: Fill in the correct volume to be administered on the measuring device.

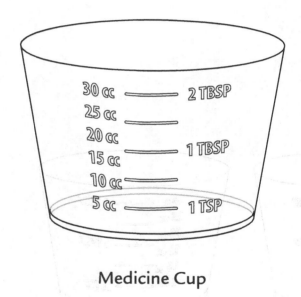

Medicine Cup

Chapter Practice Test, #11

Directions: Select the measuring device that will be used and fill in the volume to be administered with each dose.

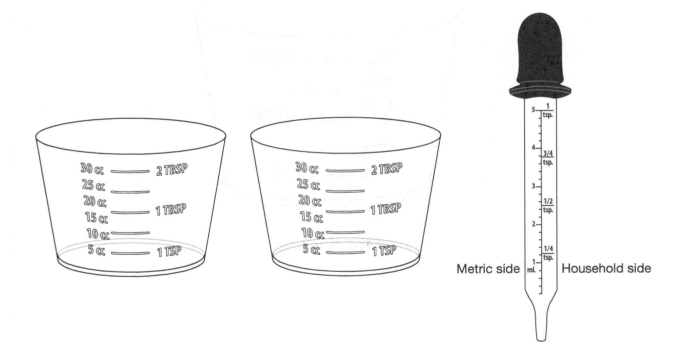

Medicine Cup   Medicine Cup   Dropper

Chapter Practice Test, #12

Directions: Select the measuring device that will be used and fill in the volume to be administered with each dose.

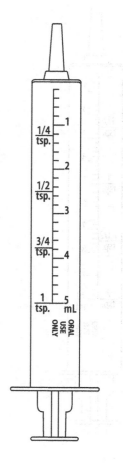

5 mL Oral Syringe

10 mL Oral Syringe

Chapter Practice Test, #18

Directions: Select the measuring device that will be used and fill in the volume to be administered with each dose.

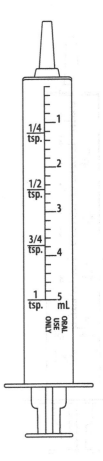

5 mL Oral Syringe

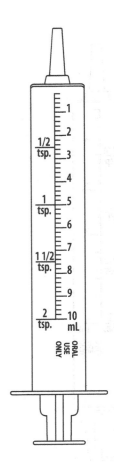

10 mL Oral Syringe

Chapter Practice Test, #19

Directions: Select the measuring device that will be used and fill in the volume to be administered with each dose.

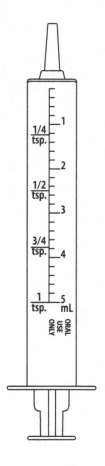

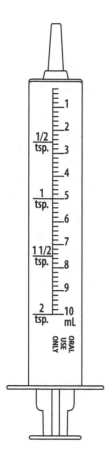

5 mL Oral Syringe   10 mL Oral Syringe

6.1 Problem Set, #1

Directions: Fill in the correct volume to be administered on the measuring device.

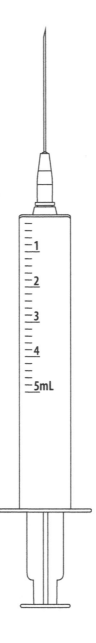

5 mL Syringe

6.1 Problem Set, #2

Directions: Fill in the correct volume to be administered on the measuring device.

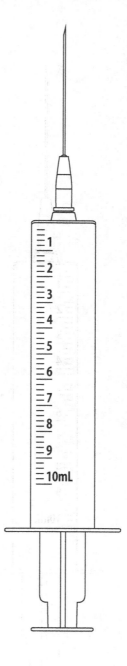

1
2
3
4
5
6
7
8
9
10mL

10 mL Syringe

6.1 Problem Set, #3

Directions: Fill in the correct volume to be administered on the measuring device.

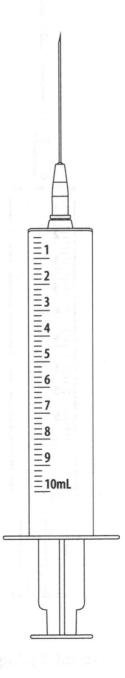

1
2
3
4
5
6
7
8
9
10mL

10 mL Syringe

6.1 Problem Set, #4

Directions: Fill in the correct volume to be administered on the measuring device.

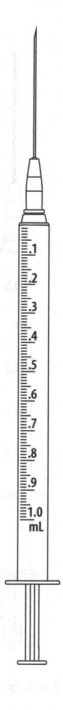

1 mL Syringe

6.1 Problem Set, #5

Directions: Fill in the correct volume to be administered on the measuring device.

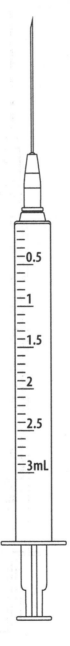

3 mL Syringe

6.1 Problem Set, #6

Directions: Fill in the correct volume to be administered on the measuring device.

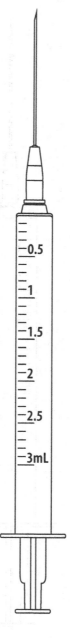

0.5
1
1.5
2
2.5
3mL

3 mL Syringe

6.1 Problem Set, #7

Directions: Fill in the correct volume to be administered on the measuring device.

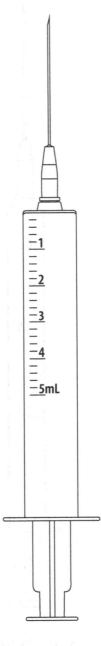

5 mL Syringe

6.1 Problem Set, #8

Directions: Fill in the correct volume to be administered on the measuring device.

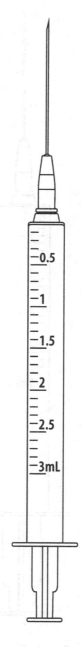

3 mL Syringe

6.1 Problem Set, #9

Directions: Fill in the correct volume to be administered on the measuring device.

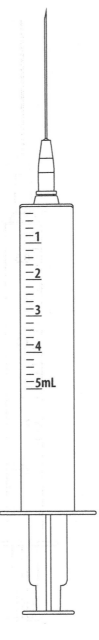

5 mL Syringe

6.1 Problem Set, #10

Directions: Fill in the correct volume to be administered on the measuring device.

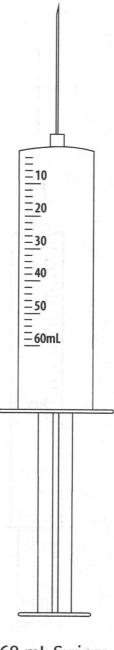

10
20
30
40
50
60mL

60 mL Syringe

6.2 Problem Set, #1

Directions: Select the measuring device that will be used and fill in the volume to be administered with each dose.

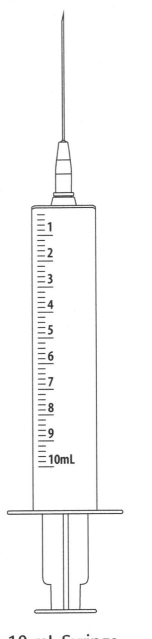

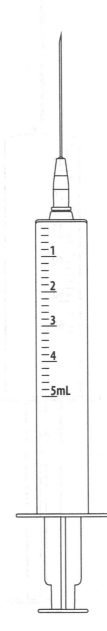

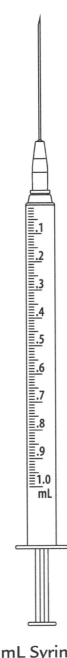

10 mL Syringe   5 mL Syringe   1 mL Syringe

6.2 Problem Set, #2

Directions: Select the measuring device that will be used and fill in the volume to be administered with each dose. You may use more than one syringe.

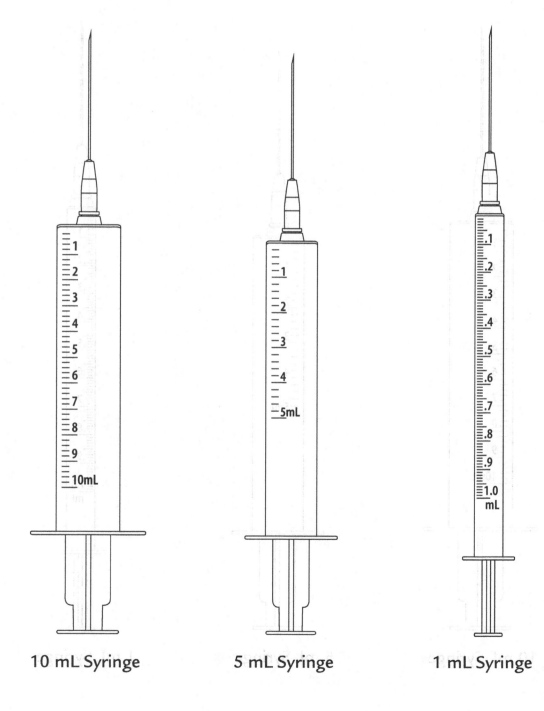

10 mL Syringe   5 mL Syringe   1 mL Syringe

6.2 Problem Set, #4

Directions: Select the measuring device that will be used and fill in the volume to be administered with each dose.

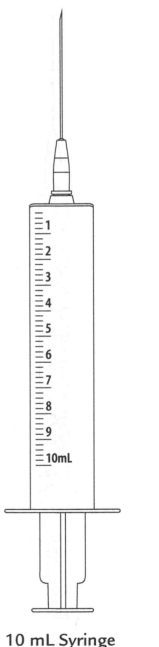

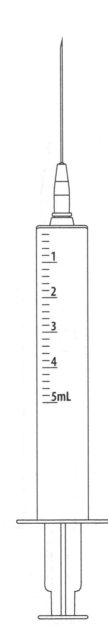

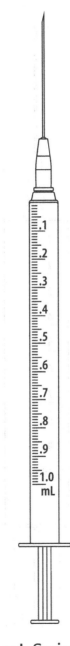

10 mL Syringe   5 mL Syringe   1 mL Syringe

6.2 Problem Set, #6

Directions: Fill in the correct volume to be administered on the measuring device.

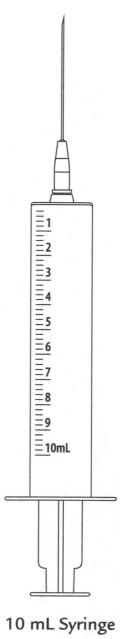

10 mL Syringe

6.2 Problem Set, #7

Directions: Select the measuring device that will be used and fill in the correct volume to be administered with each dose.

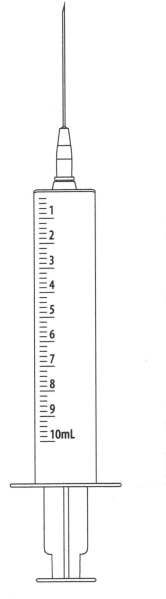

10 mL Syringe

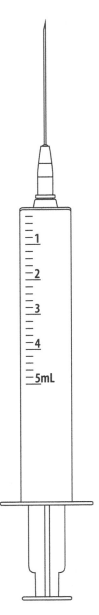

5 mL Syringe

6.2 Problem Set, #8

Directions: Fill in the correct volume to be administered on the measuring device.

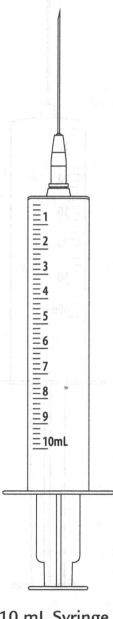

10 mL Syringe

6.2 Problem Set, #13

Directions: Fill in the correct volume to be administered on the measuring device.

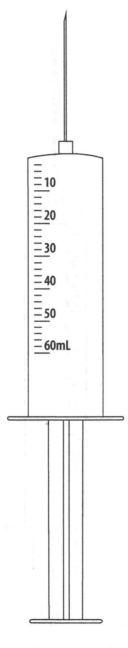

60 mL Syringe

6.2 Problem Set, #14

Directions: Fill in the correct volume to be administered on the measuring device.

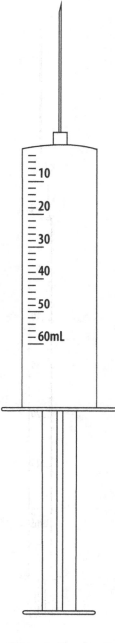

60 mL Syringe

6.2 Problem Set, #16

Directions: Fill in the correct volume to be administered on the measuring device.

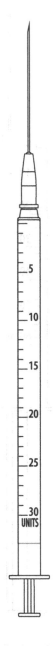

30 Unit Syringe

Finding Solutions, Scenario A, #2

Directions: Select the measuring device that will be used and fill in the volume to be administered with each dose.

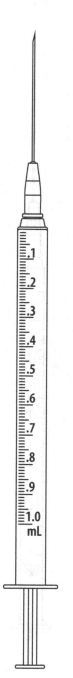

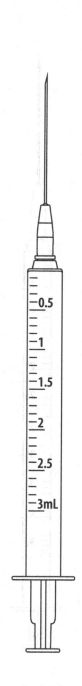

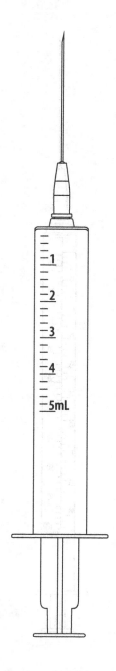

1 mL Syringe   3 mL Syringe   5 mL Syringe

Finding Solutions, Scenario B, #6 and #7

Directions: Select the measuring device that will be used and fill in the volume to be administered with each dose.

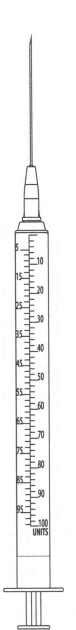

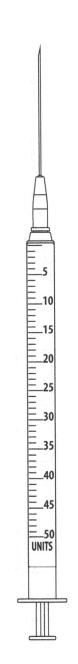

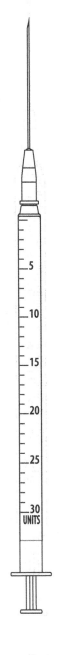

100 Unit Syringe   50 Unit Syringe   30 Unit Syringe

Chapter Practice Test, #1

Directions: Fill in the correct volume to be administered on the measuring device.

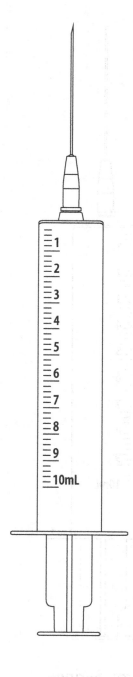

1
2
3
4
5
6
7
8
9
10mL

10 mL Syringe

Chapter Practice Test, #2

Directions: Fill in the correct volume to be administered on the measuring device.

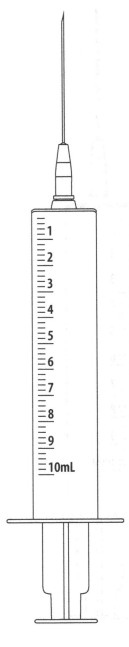

10 mL Syringe

Chapter Practice Test, #3

Directions: Fill in the correct volume to be administered on the measuring device.

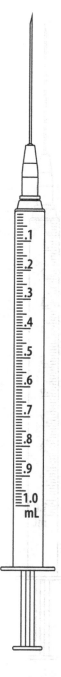

1 mL Syringe

Chapter Practice Test, #4

Directions: Fill in the correct volume to be administered on the measuring device.

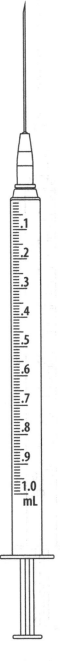

.1
.2
.3
.4
.5
.6
.7
.8
.9
1.0
mL

1 mL Syringe

Chapter Practice Test, #23

Directions: Select the measuring device that will be used and fill in the volume to be administered with each dose.

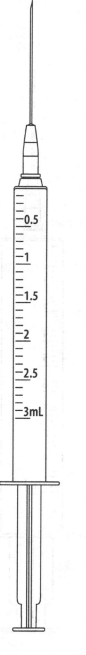

3 mL Syringe

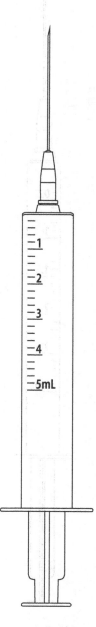

5 mL Syringe

Chapter Practice Test, #24

Directions: Select the measuring device that will be used and fill in the volume to be administered with each dose.

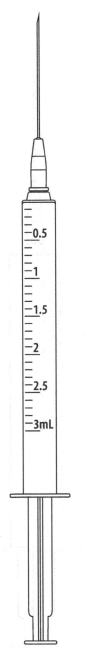

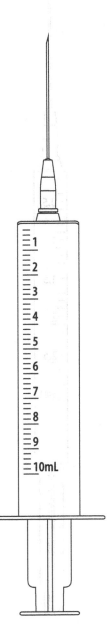

3 mL Syringe   10 mL Syringe

Chapter Practice Test, #25

Directions: Select the measuring device that will be used and fill in the volume to be administered with each dose.

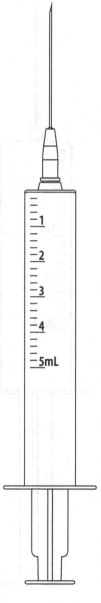

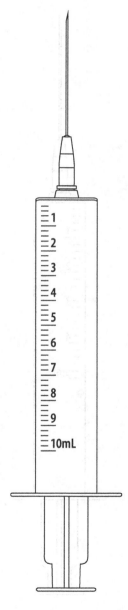

5 mL Syringe

10 mL Syringe

Chapter Practice Test, #26

Directions: Select the measuring device that will be used and fill in the volume to be administered with each dose.

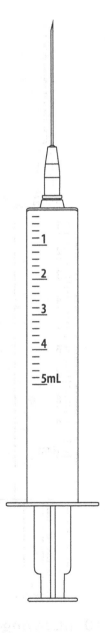

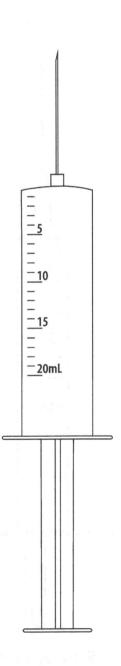

5 mL Syringe

20 mL Syringe

Chapter Practice Test, #27

Directions: Select the measuring device that will be used and fill in the volume to be administered with each dose.

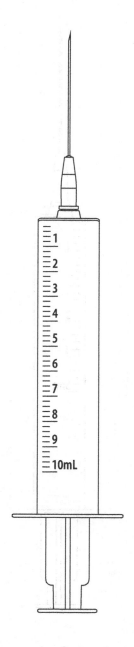

10 mL Syringe

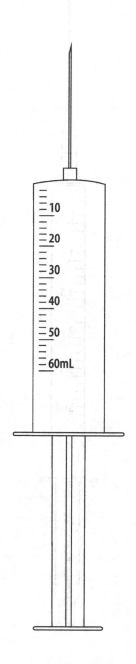

60 mL Syringe

Chapter Practice Test, #28

Directions: Select the measuring device that will be used and fill in the volume to be administered with each dose.

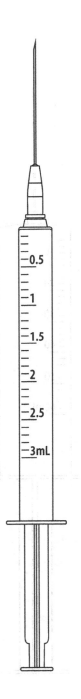

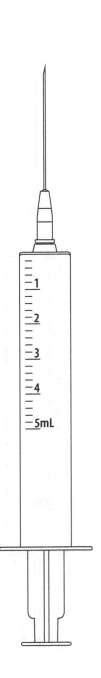

3 mL Syringe   5 mL Syringe

Chapter Practice Test, #29

Directions: Select the measuring device that will be used and fill in the volume to be administered with each dose.

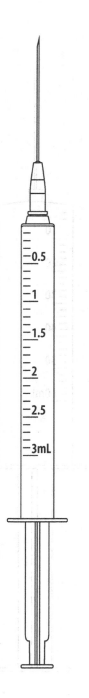

3 mL Syringe

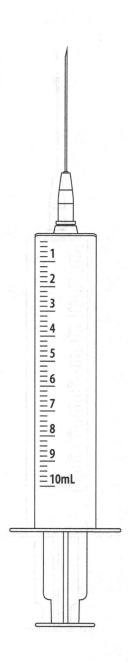

10 mL Syringe

Chapter Practice Test, #30

Directions: Select the measuring device that will be used and fill in the volume to be administered with each dose.

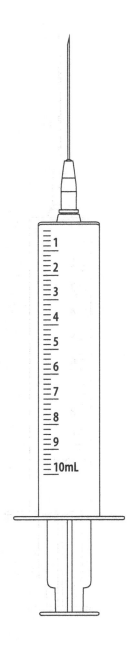

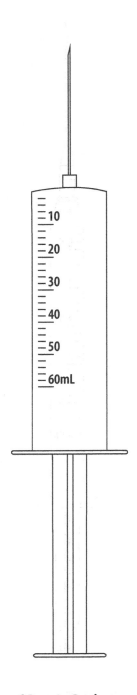

10 mL Syringe

60 mL Syringe

Chapter Practice Test, #1b

Directions: Select the measuring device that will be used and fill in the volume to be administered with each dose.

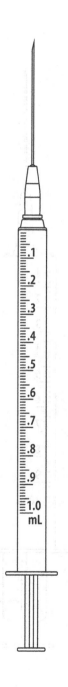

1 mL Syringe

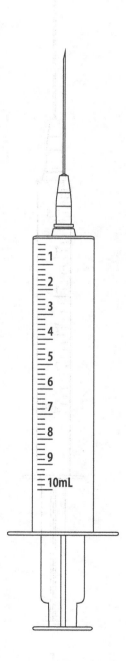

10 mL Syringe

Chapter Practice Test, #1c

Directions: Select the measuring device that will be used and fill in the volume to be administered with each dose.

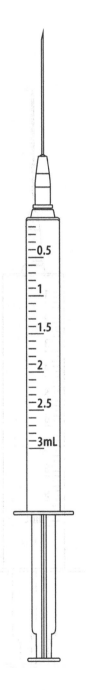

3 mL Syringe

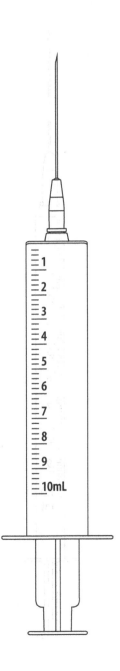

10 mL Syringe

Chapter Practice Test, #2b

Directions: Select the measuring device that will be used and fill in the volume to be administered with each dose.

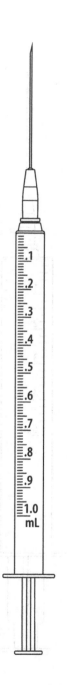

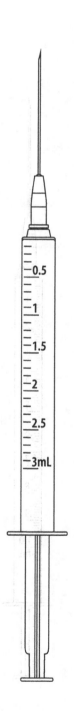

| 1 mL Syringe | 3 mL Syringe |

Chapter Practice Test, #2c

Directions: Select the measuring device that will be used and fill in the volume to be administered with each dose.

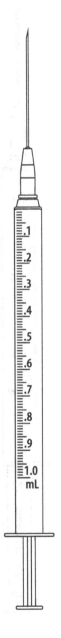

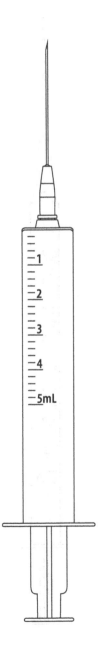

1 mL Syringe   5 mL Syringe

Chapter Practice Test, #3b

Directions: Select the measuring device that will be used and fill in the volume to be administered with each dose.

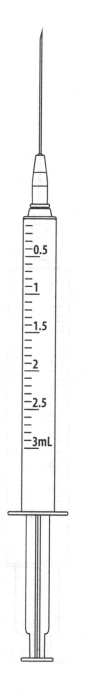

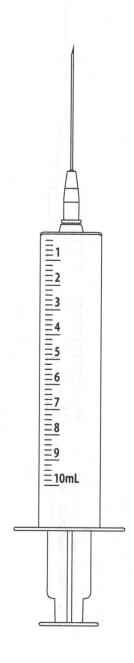

3 mL Syringe   10 mL Syringe

Chapter Practice Test, #3c

Directions: Select the measuring device that will be used and fill in the volume to be administered with each dose.

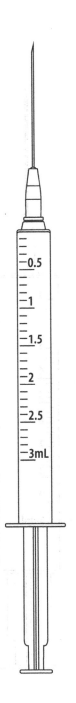

3 mL Syringe

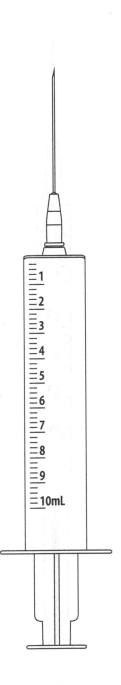

10 mL Syringe

Chapter Practice Test, #5

Directions: Select the measuring device that will be used and fill in the volume to be administered with each dose.

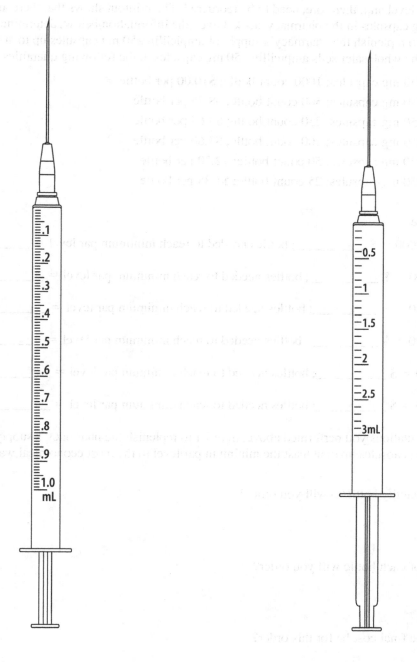

1 mL Syringe   3 mL Syringe

Finding Solutions, Scenario A, #1–#3

To gain practice in handling challenging situations in the workplace, consider the following real-world scenario and then use the guiding questions to help you formulate your responses.

Scenario A: In your pharmacy, the minimum par level for ampicillin 250 mg capsules is 500; the maximum par level is 2000. At the end of the day, the pharmacy computer prints a list of items that have fallen below the minimum par level and, therefore, need to be reordered. The printout shows that there are currently 350 ampicillin 250 mg capsules in the pharmacy stock. Given the information below, determine the most economical way to replenish the pharmacy's supply of ampicillin 250 mg capsules up to at least the minimum par level. The wholesaler sells ampicillin 250 mg capsules in the following quantities and prices:

Ampicillin 250 mg capsules; 1000 count bottle; $10.00 per bottle

Ampicillin 250 mg capsules; 500 count bottle; $8.75 per bottle

Ampicillin 250 mg capsules; 250 count bottle; $4.65 per bottle

Ampicillin 250 mg capsules; 100 count bottle; $3.60 per bottle

Ampicillin 250 mg capsules; 50 count bottle; $2.50 per bottle

Ampicillin 250 mg capsules; 25 count bottle; $1.85 per bottle

Price per capsule

$10.00/1000 = $ _____; bottles needed to reach minimum par level = _____

$8.75/500 = $ _____; bottles needed to reach minimum par level = _____

$4.65/250 = $_____; bottles needed to reach minimum par level = _____

$3.60/100 = $ _____; bottles needed to reach minimum par level =_____

$2.50/50 = $ _____; bottles needed to reach minimum par level = _____

$1.85/25 = $ _____; bottles needed to reach minimum par level = _____

Based on the calculations you performed above, in order to replenish the pharmacy's supply of ampicillin 250 mg capsules up to at least the minimum par level in the most economical way possible:

1. What size/quantity bottle(s) will you order?

2. How many of each bottle will you order?

3. What will the final cost be for this order?

Finding Solutions, Scenario B, #4–#7

To gain practice in handling challenging situations in the workplace, consider the following real-world scenario and then use the guiding questions to help you formulate your responses.

Scenario B: Beneficial HMO pays a per-client capitation fee of $149.00 per month to the Georgetown Pharmacy. The pharmacy is contracted to serve 127 of the HMO's clients and their families. During the month of December, 21 of these clients and/or their family members had a total of 52 prescriptions filled at the pharmacy. The pharmacy's total drug cost for these prescriptions was $6283.24. The contract allows the pharmacy to bill a $3.50 dispensing fee for each filled prescription.

4. What is the total amount that the HMO reimbursed the pharmacy for capitation fees?

    Monthly capitation fee = $ _____ × _____ patients = $ _____

5. What is the pharmacy's drug cost for all of the prescriptions on this plan?

    Pharmacy drug cost for 52 prescriptions for 21 patients = $_____

6. Did the pharmacy make a profit or lose money?

    Total capitation fees (from question 4) $ _____

    Pharmacy dispensing fee = $ _____ × _____ prescriptions dispensed = $ _____

    Total capitation fees $ _____ + $ _____ total dispensing fees = $ _____

7. If the pharmacy made a profit, what was the amount? If the pharmacy took a loss, what was the amount?

    Amount of profit or loss (from question 6) = $ _____

Finding Solutions, Scenario D, #9

Directions: Fill in the correct volume to be administered on the measuring device.

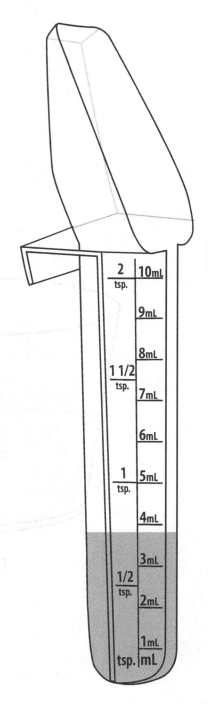

Dosing Spoon

Finding Solutions, Scenario A, #1

Directions: Select the measuring device that will be used and fill in the volume to be administered with each dose.

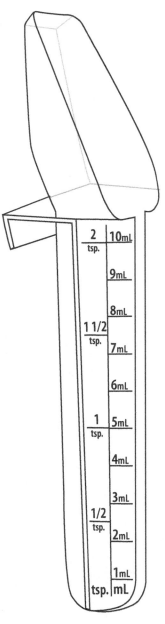

Dosing Spoon

Dosing Cup

Finding Solutions, Scenario B, #9

Directions: Select the measuring device that will be used and fill in the volume to be administered with each dose.

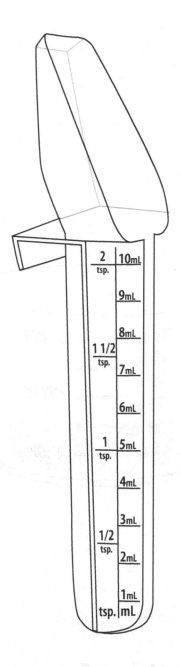

Dosing Spoon

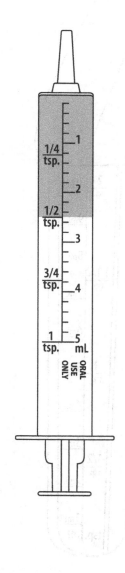

Oral Syringe

Finding Solutions, Scenario B, #10

Directions: Select the measuring device that will be used and fill in the volume to be administered with each dose.

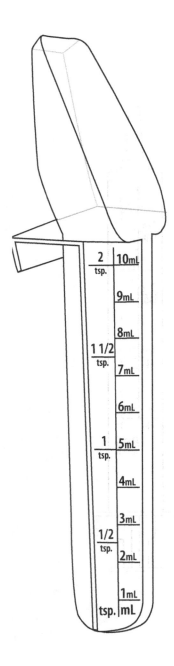

Dosing Spoon

Medicine Cup

Chapter Practice Test, #8

Directions: Select the measuring device that will be used and fill in the volume to be administered with each dose.

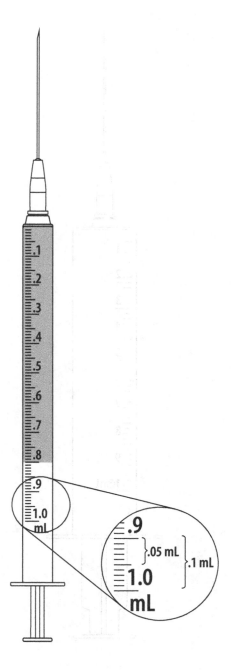

1 mL Syringe

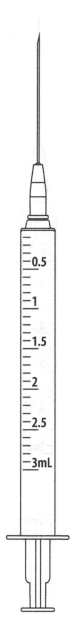

3 mL Syringe

Chapter Practice Test, #10

Directions: Select the measuring device that will be used and fill in the volume to be administered with each dose.

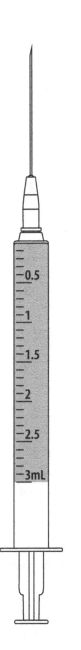

0.5
1
1.5
2
2.5
3mL

1
2
3
4
5
6
7
8
9
10mL

3 mL Syringe   10 mL Syringe

Chapter Practice Test, #14

Directions: Select the measuring device that will be used and fill in the volume to be administered with each dose.

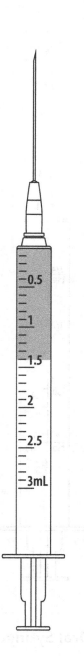

3 mL Syringe

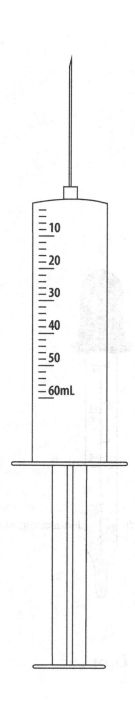

60 mL Syringe

Chapter Practice Test, #15

Directions: Select the measuring device that will be used and fill in the volume to be administered with each dose.

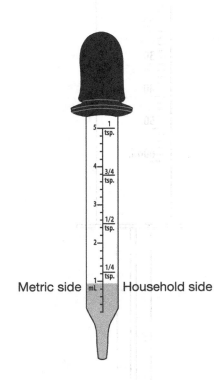

Metric side   Household side

Dropper

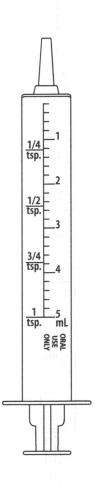

Oral Syringe

Chapter Practice Test, #16

Directions: Select the measuring device that will be used and fill in the volume to be administered with each dose.

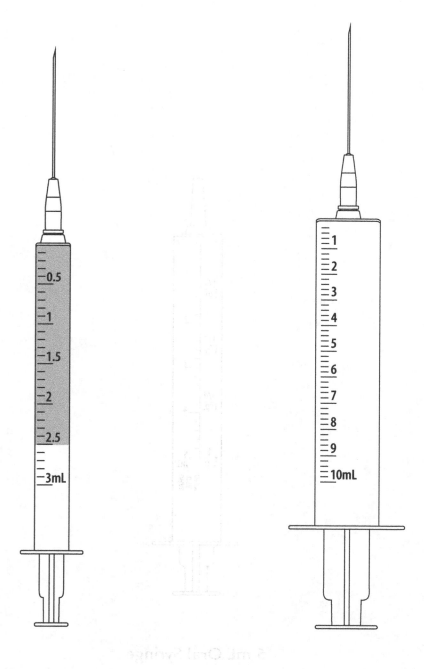

3 mL Syringe   10 mL Syringe

Finding Solutions, Scenario A, #4

Directions: Fill in the correct volume to be administered on the measuring device.

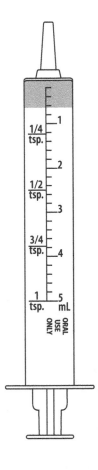

5 mL Oral Syringe

Finding Solutions, Scenario B, #8

Directions: Fill in the correct volume to be administered on the measuring device.

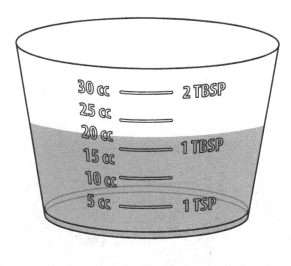

Medicine Cup

Chapter Practice Test, #11

Directions: Select the measuring device that will be used and fill in the volume to be administered with each dose.

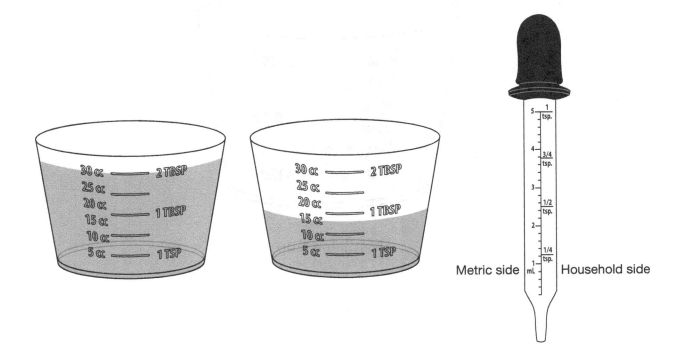

Medicine Cup   Medicine Cup   Dropper

Chapter Practice Test, #12

Directions: Select the measuring device that will be used and fill in the volume to be administered with each dose.

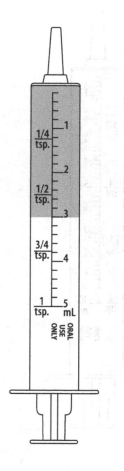

5 mL Oral Syringe   10 mL Oral Syringe

Chapter Practice Test, #18

Directions: Select the measuring device that will be used and fill in the volume to be administered with each dose.

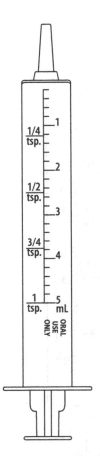

5 mL Oral Syringe

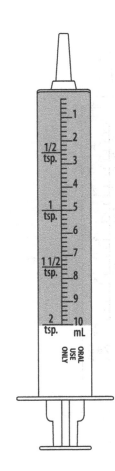

10 mL Oral Syringe

Chapter Practice Test, #19

Directions: Select the measuring device that will be used and fill in the volume to be administered with each dose.

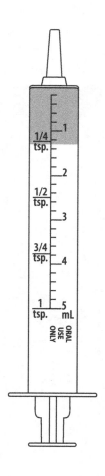

5 mL Oral Syringe   10 mL Oral Syringe

6.1 Problem Set, #1

Directions: Fill in the correct volume to be administered on the measuring device.

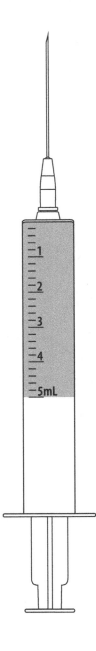

1

2

3

4

5mL

5 mL Syringe

6.1 Problem Set, #2

Directions: Fill in the correct volume to be administered on the measuring device.

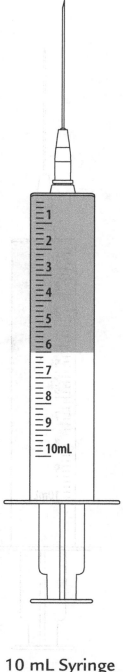

10 mL Syringe

6.1 Problem Set, #3

Directions: Fill in the correct volume to be administered on the measuring device.

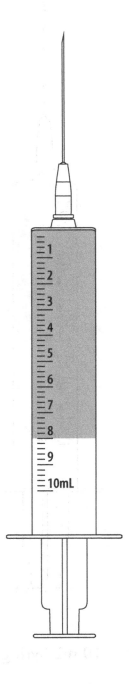

10 mL Syringe

6.1 Problem Set, #4

Directions: Fill in the correct volume to be administered on the measuring device.

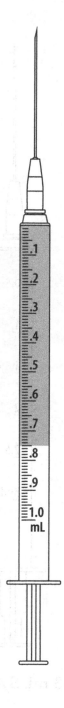

1 mL Syringe

6.1 Problem Set, #5

Directions: Fill in the correct volume to be administered on the measuring device.

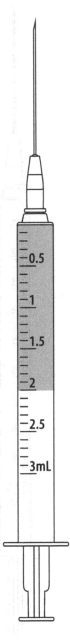

3 mL Syringe

6.1 Problem Set, #6

Directions: Fill in the correct volume to be administered on the measuring device.

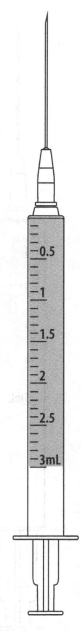

3 mL Syringe

6.1 Problem Set, #7

Directions: Fill in the correct volume to be administered on the measuring device.

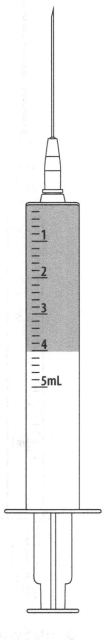

5 mL Syringe

6.1 Problem Set, #8

Directions: Fill in the correct volume to be administered on the measuring device.

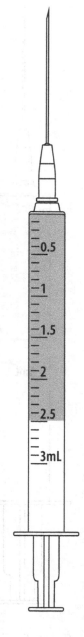

3 mL Syringe

6.1 Problem Set, #9

Directions: Fill in the correct volume to be administered on the measuring device.

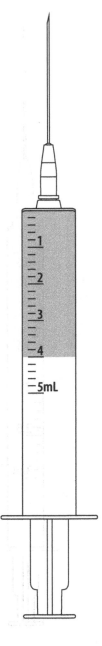

5 mL Syringe

6.1 Problem Set, #10

Directions: Fill in the correct volume to be administered on the measuring device.

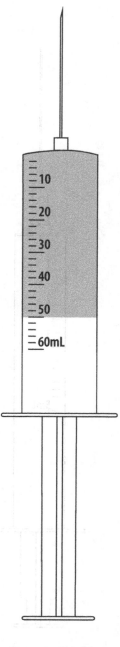

60 mL Syringe

6.2 Problem Set, #1

Directions: Select the measuring device that will be used and fill in the volume to be administered with each dose.

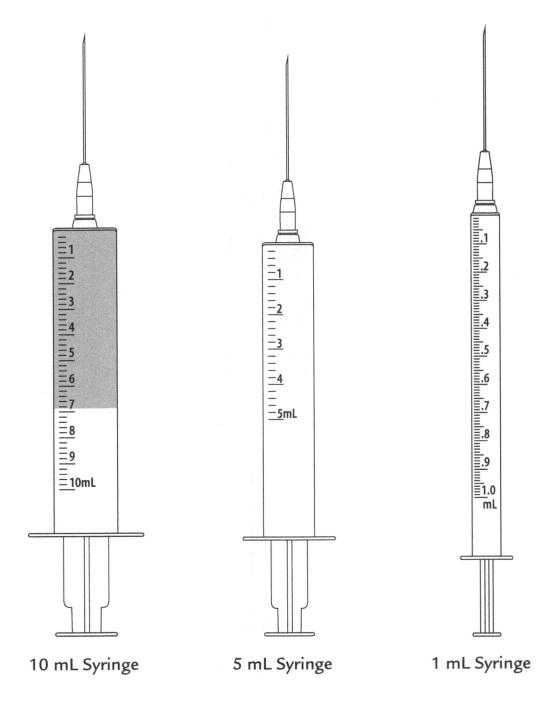

10 mL Syringe   5 mL Syringe   1 mL Syringe

6.2 Problem Set, #2

Directions: Select the measuring device that will be used and fill in the volume to be administered with each dose. You may use more than one syringe.

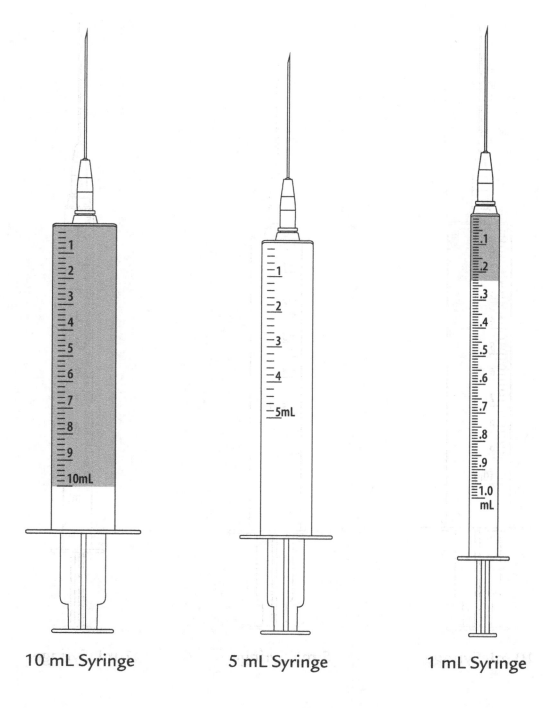

10 mL Syringe   5 mL Syringe   1 mL Syringe

6.2 Problem Set, #4

Directions: Select the measuring device that will be used and fill in the volume to be administered with each dose.

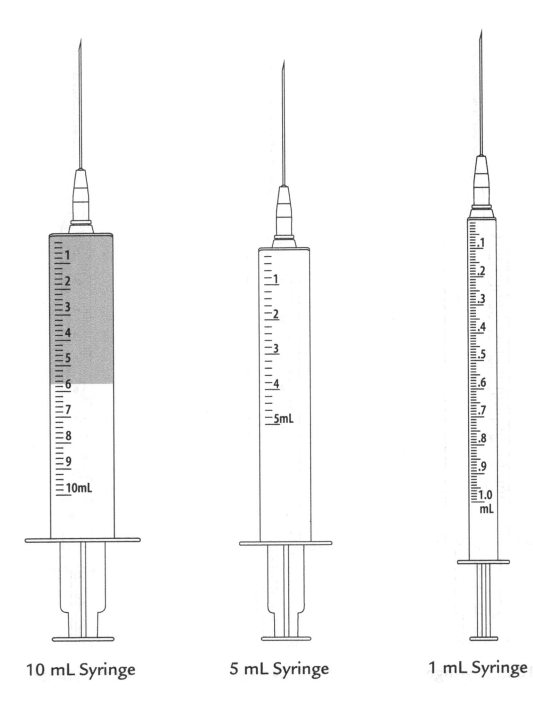

10 mL Syringe   5 mL Syringe   1 mL Syringe

6.2 Problem Set, #6

Directions: Fill in the correct volume to be administered on the measuring device.

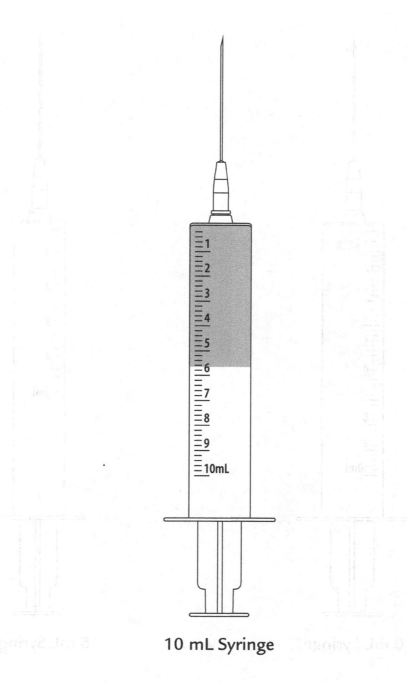

10 mL Syringe

6.2 Problem Set, #7

Directions: Select the measuring device that will be used and fill in the correct volume to be administered with each dose.

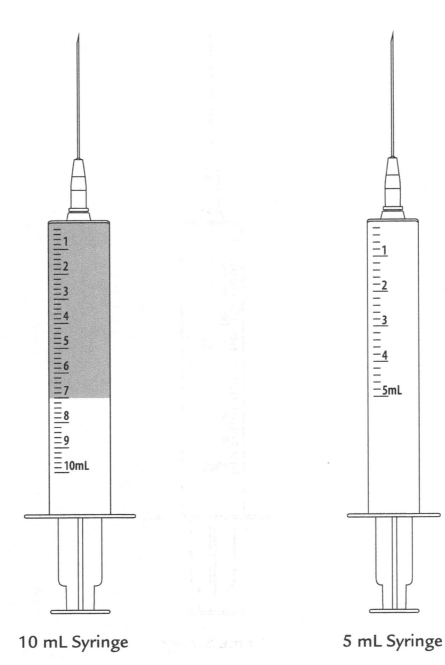

10 mL Syringe   5 mL Syringe

6.2 Problem Set, #8

Directions: Fill in the correct volume to be administered on the measuring device.

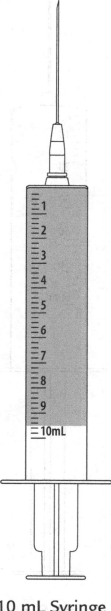

10 mL Syringe

6.2 Problem Set, #13

Directions: Fill in the correct volume to be administered on the measuring device.

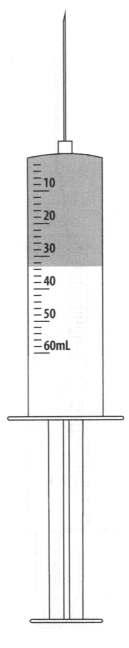

10
20
30
40
50
60mL

60 mL Syringe

6.2 Problem Set, #14

Directions: Fill in the correct volume to be administered on the measuring device.

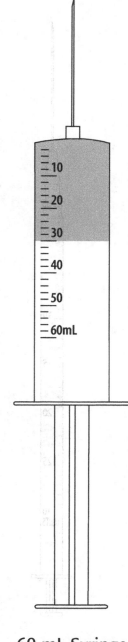

60 mL Syringe

6.2 Problem Set, #16

Directions: Fill in the correct volume to be administered on the measuring device.

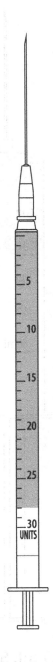

5

10

15

20

25

30
UNITS

30 Unit Syringe

Finding Solutions, Scenario A, #2

Directions: Select the measuring device that will be used and fill in the volume to be administered with each dose.

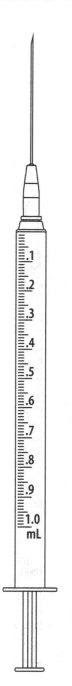

1 mL Syringe

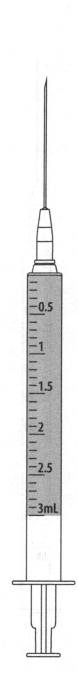

3 mL Syringe

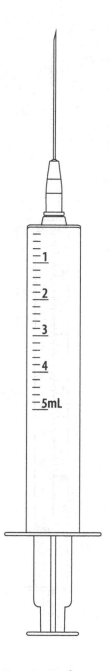

5 mL Syringe

Finding Solutions, Scenario B, #6 and #7

Directions: Select the measuring device that will be used and fill in the volume to be administered with each dose.

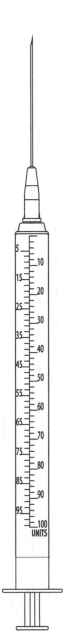

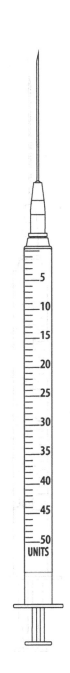

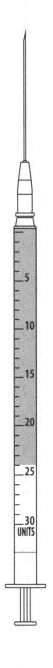

100 Unit Syringe   **50 Unit Syringe**   **30 Unit Syringe**

Chapter Practice Test, #1

Directions: Fill in the correct volume to be administered on the measuring device.

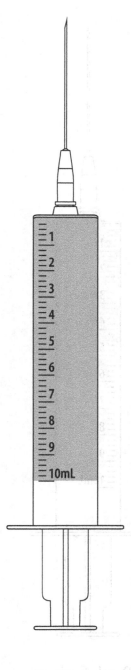

10 mL Syringe

Chapter Practice Test, #2

Directions: Fill in the correct volume to be administered on the measuring device.

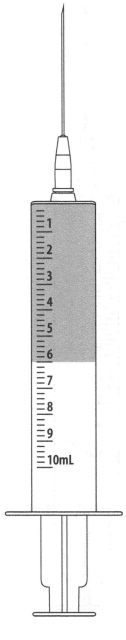

10 mL Syringe

Chapter Practice Test, #3

Directions: Fill in the correct volume to be administered on the measuring device.

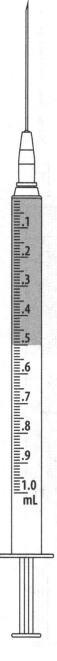

1 mL Syringe

Chapter Practice Test, #4

Directions: Fill in the correct volume to be administered on the measuring device.

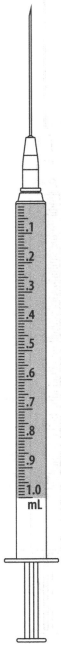

1 mL Syringe

Chapter Practice Test, #23

Directions: Select the measuring device that will be used and fill in the volume to be administered with each dose.

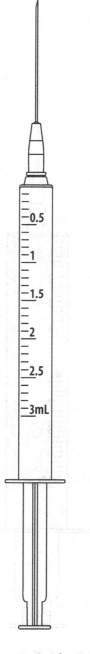

3 mL Syringe

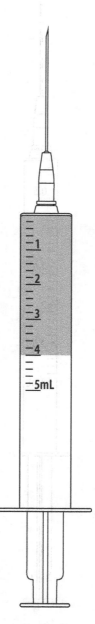

5 mL Syringe

Chapter Practice Test, #24

Directions: Select the measuring device that will be used and fill in the volume to be administered with each dose.

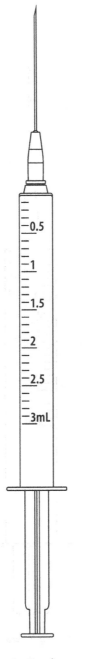

3 mL Syringe

10 mL Syringe

Chapter Practice Test, #25

Directions: Select the measuring device that will be used and fill in the volume to be administered with each dose.

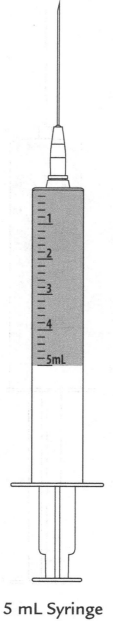

5 mL Syringe   10 mL Syringe

Chapter Practice Test, #26

Directions: Select the measuring device that will be used and fill in the volume to be administered with each dose.

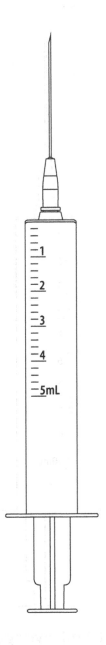

5 mL Syringe

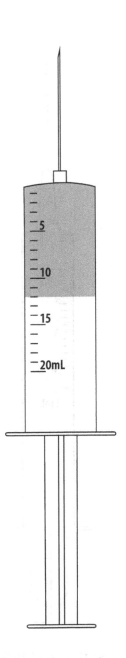

20 mL Syringe

Chapter Practice Test, #27

Directions: Select the measuring device that will be used and fill in the volume to be administered with each dose.

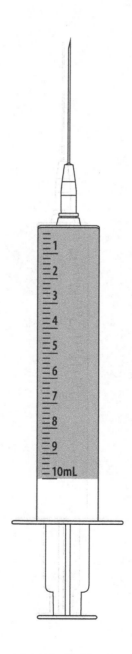

10 mL Syringe

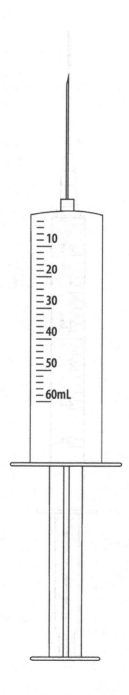

60 mL Syringe

Chapter Practice Test, #28

Directions: Select the measuring device that will be used and fill in the volume to be administered with each dose.

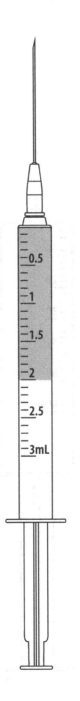

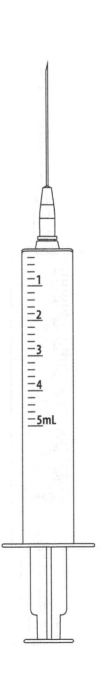

3 mL Syringe

5 mL Syringe

Chapter Practice Test, #29

Directions: Select the measuring device that will be used and fill in the volume to be administered with each dose.

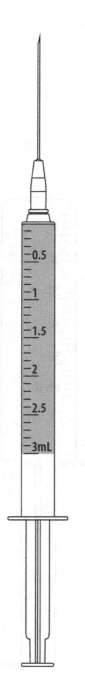

3 mL Syringe

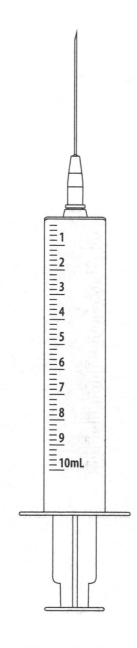

10 mL Syringe

Chapter Practice Test, #30

Directions: Select the measuring device that will be used and fill in the volume to be administered with each dose.

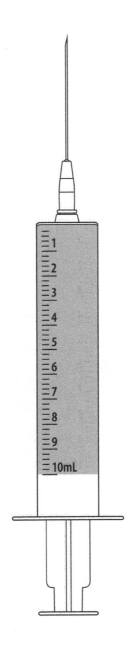

10 mL Syringe

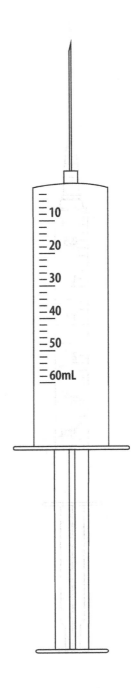

60 mL Syringe

Chapter Practice Test, #1b

Directions: Select the measuring device that will be used and fill in the volume to be administered with each dose.

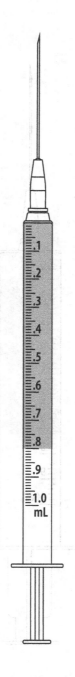

1 mL Syringe

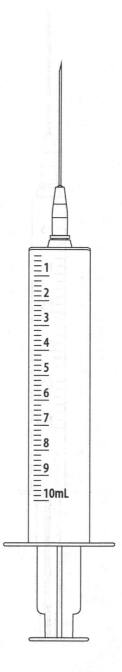

10 mL Syringe

Chapter Practice Test, #1c

Directions: Select the measuring device that will be used and fill in the volume to be administered with each dose.

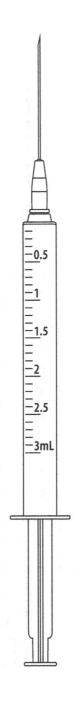

3 mL Syringe

10 mL Syringe

Chapter Practice Test, #2b

Directions: Select the measuring device that will be used and fill in the volume to be administered with each dose.

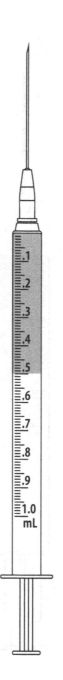

1 mL Syringe

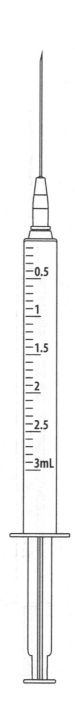

3 mL Syringe

Chapter Practice Test, #2c

Directions: Select the measuring device that will be used and fill in the volume to be administered with each dose.

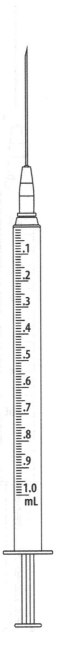

1 mL Syringe

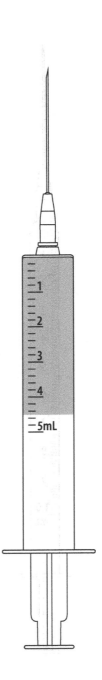

5 mL Syringe

Chapter Practice Test, #3b

Directions: Select the measuring device that will be used and fill in the volume to be administered with each dose.

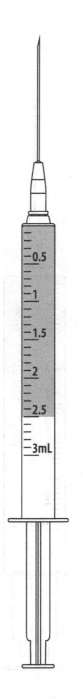

3 mL Syringe

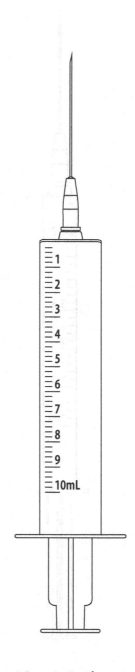

10 mL Syringe

Chapter Practice Test, #3c

Directions: Select the measuring device that will be used and fill in the volume to be administered with each dose.

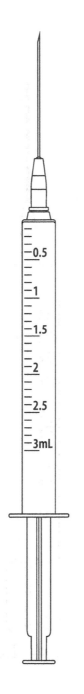

3 mL Syringe

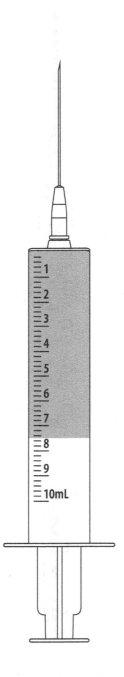

10 mL Syringe

Chapter Practice Test, #5

Directions: Select the measuring device that will be used and fill in the volume to be administered with each dose.

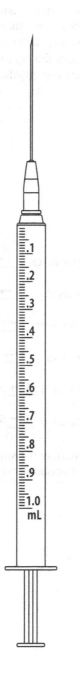

1 mL Syringe

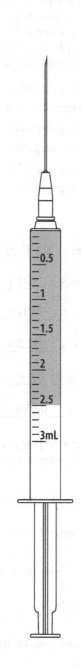

3 mL Syringe

Finding Solutions, Scenario A, #1–#3

To gain practice in handling challenging situations in the workplace, consider the following real-world scenario and then use the guiding questions to help you formulate your responses.

Scenario A: In your pharmacy, the minimum par level for ampicillin 250 mg capsules is 500; the maximum par level is 2000. At the end of the day, the pharmacy computer prints a list of items that have fallen below the minimum par level and, therefore, need to be reordered. The printout shows that there are currently 350 ampicillin 250 mg capsules in the pharmacy stock. Given the information below, determine the most economical way to replenish the pharmacy's supply of ampicillin 250 mg capsules up to at least the minimum par level. The wholesaler sells ampicillin 250 mg capsules in the following quantities and prices:

Ampicillin 250 mg capsules; 1000 count bottle; $10.00 per bottle

Ampicillin 250 mg capsules; 500 count bottle; $8.75 per bottle

Ampicillin 250 mg capsules; 250 count bottle; $4.65 per bottle

Ampicillin 250 mg capsules; 100 count bottle; $3.60 per bottle

Ampicillin 250 mg capsules; 50 count bottle; $2.50 per bottle

Ampicillin 250 mg capsules; 25 count bottle; $1.85 per bottle

Price per capsule

$10.00/1000 = $ ___0.01___; bottles needed to reach minimum par level = _1_ → 1350 capsules

$8.75/500 = $ ___0.018___; bottles needed to reach minimum par level = _1_ → 850 capsules

$4.65/250 = $___0.019___; bottles needed to reach minimum par level = _1_ → 600 capsules

$3.60/100 = $ ___0.036___; bottles needed to reach minimum par level = _2_ → 550 capsules

$2.50/50 = $ ___0.05___; bottles needed to reach minimum par level = _3_ → 500 capsules

$1.85/25 = $ ___0.074___; bottles needed to reach minimum par level = _6_ → 500 capsules

Based on the calculations you performed above, in order to replenish the pharmacy's supply of ampicillin 250 mg capsules up to at least the minimum par level in the most economical way possible:

1. What size/quantity bottle(s) will you order?

   1000-count bottle

2. How many of each bottle will you order?

   one bottle

3. What will the final cost be for this order?

   $10.00

Finding Solutions, Scenario B, #4–#7

To gain practice in handling challenging situations in the workplace, consider the following real-world scenario and then use the guiding questions to help you formulate your responses.

Scenario B: Beneficial HMO pays a per-client capitation fee of $149.00 per month to the Georgetown Pharmacy. The pharmacy is contracted to serve 127 of the HMO's clients and their families. During the month of December, 21 of these clients and/or their family members had a total of 52 prescriptions filled at the pharmacy. The pharmacy's total drug cost for these prescriptions was $6283.24. The contract allows the pharmacy to bill a $3.50 dispensing fee for each filled prescription.

4. What is the total amount that the HMO reimbursed the pharmacy for capitation fees?

   Monthly capitation fee = $ __149.00__ × __127__ patients = $ __18,923.00__

5. What is the pharmacy's drug cost for all of the prescriptions on this plan?

   Pharmacy drug cost for 52 prescriptions for 21 patients = $ __6283.24__

6. Did the pharmacy make a profit or lose money?

   Total capitation fees (from question 4) $ __18,923.00__

   Pharmacy dispensing fee = $ __3.50__ × __52__ prescriptions dispensed = $ __182.00__

   Total capitation fees $ __18,923.00__ + $ __182.00__ total dispensing fees = $ __19,105.00__

7. If the pharmacy made a profit, what was the amount? If the pharmacy took a loss, what was the amount?

   Amount of profit or loss (from question 6) = $ __12,821.76 profit__

Chapter Review Answer Keys

Chapter 1

Assessing Comprehension

1. b
2. d
3. a
4. c
5. a
6. b
7. d
8. b
9. a
10. a

Finding Solutions

1. 1 tablet
2. 45 tablets
3. 47 tablets
4. 2000 mg
5. 250 mg
6. 2250 mg
7. 3 ½ tablets
8. 11:30 AM
9. The dosing spoon should be filled to ¾ tsp or 3.75 mL.

Sampling the Certification Exam

1. b
2. c
3. c
4. b
5. b

Chapter 2

Assessing Comprehension

1. b
2. c
3. a
4. b
5. d
6. c
7. b
8. a
9. a
10. c

Finding Solutions

1. The dosing cup is the correct measuring device and should be filled to the 20 mL graduation mark.
2. 180 mL
3. two bottles
4. 4.08 kg
5. four cartons
6. $86.00
7. 96 tubes
8. $14.00
9. $3.44

Sampling the Certification Exam

1. d
2. d
3. c
4. d
5. a

Chapter 3

Assessing Comprehension

1. a
2. c
3. b
4. b
5. b
6. a
7. b
8. d
9. b
10. a

Finding Solutions

1. Checksum calculation: $4 + 2 + 9 = 15$; $4 + 3 + 2 = 9$; $2 \times 9 = 18$; $15 + 18 = 33$. The last digit is 3, but the DEA number has a 1 in the last place. The DEA number provided is not valid.

2. Take three tablets four times daily or as needed. Prescribers do not typically use "or as needed" for prescriptions because a patient may take it more frequently than the four times daily indicated.

3. Norco is the brand name, and hydrocodone APAP is the generic name. Prescribers typically do not write both brand names and generic names on a prescription.

4. Take one tablet by mouth every day in the morning for edema.

5. Take one tablet by mouth twice a day for stomach.

6. Take one tablet by mouth four times a day for five days for shingles.

7. Take one tablet by mouth three times a day for angina.

8. Take one tablet by mouth at bedtime for sleep.

9. Students should have selected the oral syringe. The 1 tsp oral syringe should be filled to the ½ tsp graduation mark.

10. Students should have selected the medicine cup. The 2 tbsp medicine cup should be filled to the 2 tsp graduation mark.

1. a
2. d
3. b
4. c
5. d

Chapter 4

Assessing Comprehension

1. d
2. d
3. c
4. b
5. c
6. c
7. a
8. a
9. b
10. c

Finding Solutions

1. $15 \text{ kg} \times 0.5 \text{ mg/kg} = 7.5 \text{ mg}$

2. $15 \text{ kg} \times 3 \text{ mg/kg} = 45 \text{ mg}$

3. $15 \text{ mg} \times 2 \text{ doses} = 30 \text{ mg}$; dose is in the appropriate range

4. $x \text{ mL}/15 \text{ mg} = 1 \text{ mL}/5 \text{ mg}$; $x \text{ mL} = 3 \text{ mL}$

5. $21.8 \text{ kg} \times 10 \text{ mg/kg} = 218 \text{ mg}$

6. $21.8 \text{ kg} \times 15 \text{ mg/kg} = 327 \text{ mg}$

7. Prescribed dose of 325 mg is in the appropriate range.

8. $x \text{ mL}/325 \text{ mg} = 5 \text{ mL}/160 \text{ mg}$; $x \text{ mL} = 10.2 \text{ mL}$

9. $^{12}/_{24} \times 600 \text{ mg} = 300 \text{ mg per dose}$

10. $^{80}/_{150} \times 600 = 320 \text{ mg per dose}$

11. $^{9}/_{21} \times 100 = 43 \text{ mg per dose}$

12. $^{62}/_{150} \times 100 = 41 \text{ mg per dose}$

Sampling the Certification Exam

1. a
2. b
3. c
4. b
5. a

Chapter 5

Assessing Comprehension

1. b
2. a
3. c
4. d
5. c

6. c
7. a
8. d
9. c
10. b

Finding Solutions

1. 22 lb $\times$ 1 kg/2.2 lb = 10 kg

2. 10 kg $\times$ 1 mg/kg = 10 mg

3. 10 mg/2 doses = 5 mg

4. x mL/5 mg $\times$ 5 mL/40 mg; x = 0.625 mL; the 5 mL oral syringe should be filled to 0.625 mL.

5. less than 1 teaspoon

6. oral syringe

7. 4 g = 4000 mg; 4000 mg divided by 4 doses = 1000 mg/dose

8. x mL/1000 mg = 5 mL/250 mg; x = 20 mL; the medicine cup should be filled to 20 mL (20 cc).

9. x tsp/20 mL = 1 tsp/5 mL; x = 4 tsp

10. 20 mL $\times$ 4 doses/day = 80 mL; 80 mL $\times$ 10 days = 800 mL

Sampling the Certification Exam

1. c
2. c
3. b

4. c
5. c

Chapter 6

Assessing Comprehension

1. c
2. b
3. b
4. d
5. a

6. b
7. a
8. b
9. a
10. d

Finding Solutions

1. x mL/100 mg = 1 mL/50 mg; x = 2 mL

2. The 3 mL syringe should be filled to the 3 mL graduation mark.

3. x mg/50 mL = 50 mg/1 mL ; x mg = 2500 mg

4. 2500 mg/100 mg dose = 25 doses

5. x units/30 days = 30 units/1 day; x units = 900 units; x mL/900 units = 1 mL/100 units; x mL = 9 mL; 1 vial will be needed

6. The 30 unit insulin syringe should be selected to deliver 30 units (equivalent to 0.3 mL).

7. 30 units − 6 units = 24 units; the 30 unit syringe should be filled to 24 units (equivalent to 0.24 mL)

Sampling the Certification Exam

1. b
2. c
3. d

4. d
5. a

Chapter 7

Assessing Comprehension

1. b
2. a
3. a
4. c
5. c

6. c
7. a
8. d
9. d
10. a

Finding Solutions

1. 20 mEq/L $\times$ 3 L = 60 mEq

2. 5 g/L $\times$ 3 L = 15 g

3. NS = 900 mg of sodium/L $\times$ 3 L = 2.7; 2.7 g in 24 hr

4. 2.5 g/500 mL = x g/480 mL = 2.4 g of dextrose

5. 1 g/500 mL = x g/480 mL = 0.96 g = 960 mg of aminophylline

6. 20 mL/1 hr = x mL/24 hr = 480 mL

Sampling the Certification Exam

1. a
2. b
3. b

4. c
5. a

Chapter 8

Assessing Comprehension

1. c
2. a
3. b
4. a
5. c

6. c
7. a
8. a
9. c
10. a

Finding Solutions

1. 20 mEq/L = 20 mEq for one bag

2. 1000/125 = 8; 24/8 = 3; 3 bags are needed for 24 hours

3. 1000 $\times$ 12 = 12,000; 12,000/50 = 240 mL of 50% dextrose

4. 1000 − 240 = 760 mL of sterile water

5. 125 mL/1 hr = x mL/24 hr; 125 $\times$ 24 = 3000 mL; the patient will receive 3000 mL of IV fluid in 24 hours

6. 150 mL/1 hr = x mL/24 hr; 150 $\times$ 24 = 3600 mL; 3600/1 = 3600; 3600 mL will be needed for 24 hours

7. 3600 $\times$ 15 = 54,000; 54,000/70 = 771.43 mL of D70%

8. 3600 $\times$ 5 = 18,000; 18,000/10 = 1800 mL of AA 10%

9. 3600 $\times$ 2.5 = 9000; 9000/10 = 900 mL of Liposyn 10%

10. 10 mEq/1000 mL = x mEq/3600 mL; 36,000/1000 = 36 mEq/bag

    4 mEq/1 mL = 36 mEq/x mL; 1 $\times$ 36 = 36; 36/4 = 9 mL of NaCl

11. 10 mEq/1000 mL = x mEq/3600 mL; 10 $\times$ 3600 = 36,000/1000 = 36 mEq/bag

    2 mEq/1 mL = 36 mEq/x mL; 1 $\times$ 36 = 36; 36/2 = 18 mL of KCl

12. 2.5 mEq/1000 mL = x mEq/3600 mL; 2.5 $\times$ 3600 = 9000; 9000/1000 = 9 mEq/bag

    4.06 mEq/1 mL = 9 mEq/x mL; 1 $\times$ 90 = 9; 9/4.06 = 2.22 mL of $MgSO_4$

13. 20 units/1000 mL = x units/3600 mL; 20 $\times$ 3600 = 72,000; 72,000/1000 mL = 72 units/bag

    100 units/1 mL = 72 units/x mL; 1 $\times$ 72 = 72; 72/100 = 0.72 mL of insulin

14. 10 mL of MVI

15. 771.43 + 1800.00 + 900.00 + 9.00 + 18.00 + 2.22 + 0.72 + 10.00 = 3511.37

    3600 − 3511.37 = 88.63 mL of sterile water

Sampling the Certification Exam

1. b
2. b
3. b

4. d
5. b

Chapter 9

Assessing Comprehension

1. d
2. d
3. b
4. c
5. c

6. a
7. c
8. c
9. d
10. a

Finding Solutions

1. 1000-count bottle at $10.00 per bottle = $0.01 per capsule

2. one bottle

3. $10.00

4. $149.00 × 127 = $18,923.00; $3.50 × 52 = $182.00; $18,923.00 + $182.00 = $19,105.00 The amount the HMO reimbursed the pharmacy was $19,105.00.

5. $6283.24

6. The pharmacy made a profit.

7. $19,105.00 − $6283.24 = $12,821.76; the pharmacy made a profit of $12,821.76.

Sampling the Certification Exam

1. c
2. c
3. b

4. a
5. b

Chapter Practice Test Answer Keys

Chapter 1

1. ⅘
2. ¹/₁₀₀
3. 0.2
4. 0.875
5. 39
6. 216
7. MCC
8. CDLXXIII
9. 910,000,000
10. 720
11. 0.00002538
12. 0.000201
13. 3.7594×10^{11}
14. 1.09×10^{-7}
15. 1.8×10^{6}
16. 9.2×10^{2}
17. 0.91
18. 0.33
19. Tenths
20. Hundredths
21. Thousandths
22. Tens
23. 1090.6
24. 12.009647
25. 48.47
26. 13.17
27. 19.6992
28. 45.37944
29. 46
30. 12,917
31. 6.5
32. 84.0
33. 643.731
34. 4.262
35. 1.89
36. 0.7952
37. 89.5%
38. 85.0%
39. 1030
40. 1950
41. 0025
42. Estimate 140 mL; choose 240 mL size
43. Estimate $160; actual $158.47
44. 6:00 PM
45. 0700–0830

Chapter 2

1. 10 mg:1 tablet
2. 250 mg:5 mL
3. 12.5 mg:5 mL
4. 500 mg:2 mL
5. 1; 10; 100
6. 1; 100; 2.5
7. ⅛
8. ⅔
9. 0.005
10. 0.93
11. 20% solution
12. 0.4% solution
13. 0.12 g
14. 1.8 g
15. 50 tablets
16. 1.5 mL
17. 5.54%
18. 7.06%
19. 1.46%
20. 6.67%
21. a. 4.8%; b. no

22. a. 14%; b. no
23. 462.33 mL to 471.67 mL
24. 29.93 g to 30.08 g

Chapter 3

1. Meets validity
2. Meets validity
3. Meets validity
4. Does not meet validity due to checksum failure
5. 90 tablets
6. 30 tablets
7. 30 capsules or caplets
8. 30 fluid ounces
9. 90 tablets
10. 180 capsules or caplets
11. Brand/trade name: none given
    Generic name: sertraline
    Dosage form: tablets
    Strength: 100 mg
    Total quantity: 100 tablets
    Storage requirements: Store at controlled room temperature (68–77 °F)
    Manufacturer: Mylan
    NDC number: 0378-8127-01
12. Brand/trade name: Apriso
    Generic name: mesalamine
    Dosage form: (extended-release) capsules
    Strength: 0.375 g
    Total quantity: 120 capsules
    Storage requirements: Store at controlled room temperature (68–77 °F)
    Manufacturer: Salix
    NDC number: 65649-10302
13. Capsule or caplet
14. Dispense as written
15. Grain
16. Intramuscular
17. Intravenous
18. Milliliter
19. No known allergies
20. By mouth
21. Every six hours
22. Immediately
23. qs
24. ud
25. D/C
26. qid
27. g
28. L
29. mEq
30. npo
31. tab
32. c̄
33. Take one tablet by mouth every two hours as needed.
34. Instill two drops into the right eye twice daily.
35. Apply one patch topically every seven days.
36. Take one capsule by mouth three times daily before meals as directed.
37. Apply to rash as needed for itch.
38. Take one tablet by mouth every morning with food.
39. Quantity to dispense, route of administration, and DOB
40. Sig, dosage form, route of administration, and DOB
41. Apply one patch topically every 72 hours. Dispense 10 patches.
42. Take two capsules by mouth three times daily for 10 days. Dispense 60 capsules.
43. Instill one drop into the left eye twice daily for seven days. Dispense one 5 mL bottle.
44. 10 mL × 3 daily × 10 days = 300 mL. Two bottles will be needed to fill the order because there are only 240 mL in one bottle.
45. A dosing schedule refers to how often the drug is to be taken.
46. Routes of administration include any of the following: oral, injection, topical, inhalation, parenteral, transmucosal.

Chapter 4

1. 1.821 mg
2. 6.864 g
3. 34,500 mcg
4. 0.186 kg
5. 9 capsules

6. 12 doses

7. 6 tablets

8. 0.8 mL (The 1 mL syringe should be filled to the 0.8 mL graduation mark.)

9. 700 mL

10. 3 mL (The 3 mL syringe should be filled to the 3 mL graduation mark.)

11. 1120 mcg

12. 18 doses

13. 66,666.6 rounded to 66,670 mcg

14. 1.4 mL (The 3 mL syringe should be filled to the 1.4 mL graduation mark.)

15. 0.9 mL (The dropper should be filled to the 0.9 mL graduation mark.)

16. 2.5 mL (The 3 mL syringe should be filled to the 2.5 mL graduation mark.)

17. 168 mg/dose

18. Using 0.57 m(2); 0.285 mg/day

19. 9.65 mg/dose

20. Using 1.84 m(2); 230 mg

Chapter 5

1. 3 tsp × 1 tbsp/3 tsp = 1 tbsp; 1 tbsp × 1 fl oz/2 tbsp = 0.5 fl oz (½ fl oz)

2. 8 fl oz × 2 tbsp/1 fl oz = 16 tbsp; 16 tbsp × 3 tsp/1 tbsp = 48 tsp

3. 8 mL × 1 tsp/5 mL = 1.6 tsp (1⅗ tsp)

4. 8 fl oz × 30 mL/1 fl oz = 240 mL

5. 192 lb × 1 kg/2.2 lb = 87.272 kg, rounded to 87.3 kg

6. 5 fl oz = 150 mL; 150 mL × 1 dose/5 mL = 30 doses

7. 3 tsp = 15 mL; 500 mL × 1 dose/15 mL = 33.3 doses

8. 80 mg

9. 120 mg

10. x mg/150 mL = 250 mg/5 mL; x mg = 7500 mg; 7500 mg × 1 g/1000 mg = 7.5 g

11. 3 tbsp = 45 mL; x mg/45 mL = 80 mg/15 mL; x mg = 240 mg (Both medicine cups should be filled: one to the 30 mL [30 cc] graduation mark and one to the 15 mL [15 cc] graduation mark.)

12. x mg/3 mL = 10 mg/1 mL; x mg = 30 mg (The 5 mL oral syringe should be filled to the 3 mL graduation mark.)

13. x mg/12.5 mL = 125 mg/5 mL; x mg = 312.5 mg

14. 6 tsp daily = 30 mL; x days/100 mL = 1 day/30 mL; x days = 3.33 days

15. (8 tablets × 2 days) + (7 tablets × 1 day) + (6 tablets × 2 days) + (5 tablets × 1 day) + (4 tablets × 2 days) + (3 tablets × 1 day) + (2 tablets × 2 days) + (1 tablet × 1 day) + (0.5 tablet × 2 days) = 57 tablets

16. ½ tsp = 0.5 tsp = 2.5 mL; 2.5 mL × 20 mg/5 mL = 10 mg

17. ¾ tsp = 0.75 tsp = 3.75 mL; 3.75 mL × 20 mg/5 mL = 15 mg

18. 40 mg × 5 mL/20 mg = 10 mL (The 10 mL oral syringe should be filled to the 10 mL graduation mark or 2 tsp.)

19. 5 mg × 5 mL/20 mg = 1.25 mL (The 5 mL oral syringe should be filled to the 1.25 mL graduation mark.)

20. a. (43° − 32°)/1.8 = 6.111°C, rounded to 6.1 °C

    b. (40° − 32°)/1.8 = 4.44444 °C, rounded to 4.4 °C

    c. (41° − 32°)/1.8 = 5 °C

    d. (38° − 32°)/1.8 = 3.3333 °C, rounded to 3.3 °C

    e. (39° − 32°)/1.8 = 3.88888 °C, rounded to 3.9 °C

    f. (40.5° − 32°)/1.8 = 4.72222 °C, rounded to 4.7 °C

    g. (37° − 32°)/1.8 = 2.7777 °C, rounded to 2.8 °C

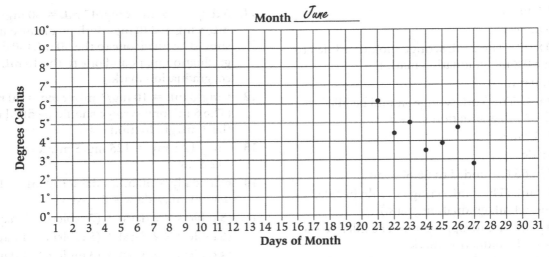

Month __June__

Degrees Celsius / Days of Month

Chapter 6

1. x mL/2 g = 5 mL/1 g; x mL = 10 mL (The 10 mL syringe should be filled to the 10 mL graduation mark.)

2. x mL/60 mg = 10 mL/100 mg; x mL = 6 mL (The 10 mL syringe should be filled to the 6 mL graduation mark.)

3. x mL/25 mg = 1 mL/50 mg; x mL = 0.5 mL (The 1 mL syringe should be filled to the 0.5 mL graduation mark.)

4. x mL/10 mg = 2 mL/20 mg; x mL = 1 mL (The 1 mL syringe should be filled to the 1 mL graduation mark.)

5. x mg/1.4 mL = 60 mg/2 mL; x mg = 42 mg

6. x mg/3.1 mL = 20 mg/1 mL; x mg = 62 mg

7. x mg/0.8 mL = 2 mg/2 mL; x mg = 0.8 mg

8. x mg/1.8 mL = 50 mg/1 mL; x mg = 90 mg

9. x g/600 mL = 1 g/200 mL; x g = 3 g

10. x mg/5 mL = 1000 mg/5000 mL; x mg = 1 mg

11. x mg/0.5 mL = 1000 mg/1000 mL; x mg = 0.5 mg

12. x mcg/0.5 mL = 1,000,000 mcg/1000 mL; x mcg = 500 mcg

13. x mL/120 mg = 1 mL/20 mg; x mL = 6 mL lidocaine
    x mL/500 mg = 10 mL/100 mg; x mL = 50 mL furosemide

14. x mL/24 mEq = 1 mL/2 mEq; x mL = 12 mL

15. a. x mL/40 g = 100 mL/5 g; x mL = 800 mL of 5%
    b. x mL/40 g = 100 mL/20 g; x mL = 200 mL of 20%

c. x mL/24 mEq = 1 mL/4 mEq; x mL = 6 mL

d. x mL/10 mEq = 1 mL/2 mEq; x mL = 5 mL

e. x mL/300 mg = 1 mL/25 mg; x mL = 12 mL

f. x mL/2 units = 1 mL/100 units; x mL = 0.02 mL

16. a. x mL/18 mEq = 1 mL/4 mEq; x mL = 4.5 mL
    b. x mL/30 mEq = 20 mL/40 mEq; x mL = 15 mL
    c. x mL/1000 mg = 1 mL/500 mg; x mL = 2 mL
    d. x mL/100 mg = 1 mL/50 mg; x mL = 2 mL

17. x mL/230,000 units = 1 mL/500,000 units; x mL = 0.46 mL

18. x mL/15,000 units = 1 mL/10,000 units; x mL = 1.5 mL

19. x mEq/3.5 mL = 4 mEq/1 mL; x mEq = 14 mEq

20. x mL/35 mg = 0.8 mL/80 mg; x mL = 0.35 mL

21. x units/0.42 mL = 100 units/1 mL; x units = 42 units

22. number of units per day: 18 units/dose × 2 doses/day = 36 units/day

    number of units in 1 vial: x units/10 mL = 100 units/1 mL; x units = 1000 units

    number of days 2 vials will last: x days/2000 units = 1 day/36 units; x days = 55.55 days, rounded to 55 days

23. Use the 20 mEq vial; x mL/16 mEq = 10 mL/20 mEq; x mL = 8 mL

24. Use the 40 mEq vial; x mL/38 mEq = 20 mL/40 mEq; x mL = 19 mL

25. 10 mL − 9.6 mL = 0.4 mL

26. x mL/2000 mg = 5 mL/150 mg; x mL = 66.7 mL; 66.7 mL − 39 mL = 27.7 mL

27. x mL/10,000 mg = 1 mL/100 mg; x mL = 100 mL; 100 mL − 87 mL = 13 mL PV; x mL/10,000 mg = 1 mL/50 mg; x mL = 200 mL; 200 mL − 13 mL = 187 mL

28. x mL/4000 mg = 5 mL/250 mg; x mL = 80 mL; 80 mL − 11.3 mL = 68.7 mL

29. 76 mL + 12.6 mL = 88.6 mL FV; x mg/1 mL = 30,000 mg/88.6 mL; x mg = 338.6 mg, so 338.6 mg/mL

30. x mL/1000 mg = 1 mL/100 mg; x mL = 10 mL; 10 mL − 8.9 mL = 1.1 mL

Chapter 7

1. 0.25 mL/100 mL
2. 3 g/100 mL
3. 10%
4. 8%
5. 10%
6. 1%
7. 27 g
8. 800 mg
9. 8 hr
10. Approximately 1:40 PM
11. 8.33 mL/min
12. 8 PM
13. a. approximately 166.67 mL/hr
    b. approximately 1333.33 mg/hr
14. a. 62.5 mL/hr
    b. 125 mg/hr
15. a. 97.5 mL/hr
    b. 19.5 mg/hr
16. 20 gtts/min
17. 10 gtts/min
18. 33.33, rounded to 33 gtts/min
19. approximately 2.3 L
20. approximately 5.56 hr or 5 hr and 33 min
21. 50 gtts/min
22. 66.66, rounded to 66 gtts/min

23. a. 4 mL (The 5 mL syringe should be filled to the 4 mL graduation mark.)
    b. approximately 100 mL/hr
24. a. 10 mL (The 10 mL syringe should be filled to the 10 mL graduation mark.)
    b. 250 gtts/min
25. a. 5 mL (The 5 mL syringe should be filled to the 5 mL graduation mark.)
    b. 83 gtts/min
26. a. 12 mL (The 20 mL syringe should be filled to the 12 mL graduation mark.
    b. approximately 100 mL/hr
27. a. 10 mL (The 10 mL syringe should be filled to the 10 mL graduation mark.)
    b. 33 gtts/min
28. a. 2 mL (The 3 mL syringe should be filled to the 2 mL graduation mark.)
    b. 10 gtts/min
29. a. 3 mL (The 3 mL syringe should be filled to the 3 mL graduation mark.)
    b. 100 gtts/min
30. a. 10 mL (The 10 mL syringe should be filled to the 10 mL graduation mark.)
    b. 40 mg/hr

Chapter 8

1. a. 5 mg/1 mL = x mg/8 mL; 5 × 8 = 40; 40/1 = 40 mg of hydrocortisone
   b. 100 mg/2 mL = 40 mg/x mL; 2 × 40 = 80; 80/100 = 0.8 mL of hydrocortisone stock solution (The 1 mL syringe should be filled to the 0.8 mL graduation mark.)
   c. 8 − 0.8 = 7.2 mL of sterile water (The 10 mL syringe should be filled to the 7.2 mL graduation mark.)
2. a. 5 mcg/1 mL = x mcg/5 mL; 5 × 5 = 25; 25/1 = 25 mcg of dopamine
   b. 50 mcg/1 mL = 25 mcg/x mL; 1 × 25 = 25; 25/50 = 0.5 mL of dopamine stock solution (The 1 mL syringe should be filled to the 0.5 mL graduation mark.)
   c. 5 − 0.5 = 4.5 mL of sterile water (The 5 mL syringe should be filled to the 4.5 graduation mark.)
3. a. 1 mg/1 mL = x mg/10 mL; 1 × 10 = 10; 10/1 = 10 mg of dexamethasone
   b. 4 mg/1 mL = 10 mg/x mL; 1 × 10 = 10; 10/4 = 2.5 mL of dexamethasone stock

solution (The 3 mL syringe should be filled to the 2.5 mL graduation mark.)

   c. $10 - 2.5 = 7.5$ mL of sterile water (The 10 mL syringe should be filled to the 7.5 mL graduation mark.)

4. 1 mg/1 mL = x mg/10 mL; $1 \times 10 = 10$; $10/1 = 10$ mg of dexamethasone

5. 1 mg/1 mL = 2.5 mg/x mL; $1 \times 2.5 = 2.5$; $2.5/1 = 2.5$ mL of the special dilution (The 3 mL syringe should be filled to the 2.5 mL graduation mark.)

6. $50\text{ g}/30\text{ g} = 1.67$
Coal tar 2 g; $2/1.67 = 1.19$; coal tar 1.19 g
Salicylic acid 0.5 g; $0.5/1.67 = 0.3$; salicylic acid 0.3 g
Triamcinolone 0.1% ung 7.5 g; $7.5/1.67 = 4.49$; triamcinolone 0.1% ung 4.49 g
Aqua-base ointment QSAD 50 g; aqua-base ointment QSAD 30 g

7. $30/10 = 3/1$
Progesterone 2.4 g; $2.4/3 = 0.8$; progesterone 0.8 g
Polyethylene glycol 3350 30 g; $30/3 = 10$; polyethylene glycol 3350 10 g
Polyethylene glycol 1000 90 g; $90/3 = 30$; polyethylene glycol 1000 30 g

8. $250/100 = 2.5/1$
Podophyllum resin 25%; 25% = 25 g $\times$ 2.5 = 62.5 g; podophyllum resin 62.5 g
Benzoin tincture QSAD 250 mL

9. $200/500 = 0.4$
Iodine 30 g; $30 \times 0.4 = 12$; iodine 12 g
Sodium iodide 25 g; $25 \times 0.4 = 10$; sodium iodide 10 g
Purified water QSAD 500 mL; purified water QSAD 200 mL

10. $120/30 = 4/1$
Antipyrine 1.8 g; $1.8 \times 4 = 7.2$; antipyrine 7.2 g
Benzocaine 0.5 g; $0.5 \times 4 = 2$; benzocaine 2 g
Glycerin QSAD 30 mL; $30 \times 4 = 120$; glycerin QSAD 120 mL

11.

10		2.5 parts of 10%
	7.5	
5		2.5 parts of 5%

$2.5 + 2.5 = 5$ parts total
$2.5/5 = x/400 = 2.5 \times 400 = 1000$; $1000/5 = 200$; 200 mL of D10%
$2.5/5 = x/400 \times 2.5 \times 400 = 1000$; $1000/5 = 200$; 200 mL of D5%

12.

20		3 parts of 20%
	8	
5		12 parts of 5%

$3 + 12 = 15$ parts total
$3/15 = x/800 = 3 \times 800 = 2400$; $2400/15 = 160$; 160 mL of D20%
$12/15 = x/800 = 12 \times 800 = 9600$; $9600/15 = 640$; 640 mL of D5%

13.

20		4 parts of 20%
	9	
5		11 parts of 5%

$4 + 11 = 15$ parts total
$4/15 = x/1000 = 4 \times 1000 = 4000$; $4000/15 = 266.66$; 266.66 mL of D20%
$11/15 = x/1000 = 11 \times 1000 = 11,000$; $11,000/15 = 733.33$ mL of D5%

14.

20		2 parts of 20%
	12	
10		8 parts of 10%

$2 + 8 = 10$ parts total
$2/10 = x/200$; $2 \times 200 = 400$; $400/10 = 40$; 40 mL of D20%
$8/10 = x/200$; $8 \times 200 = 1600$; $1600/10 = 160$ mL of D10%

15.

50		10 parts of 50%
	15	
5		35 parts of 5%

$10 + 35 = 45$ parts total

$10/45 = x/500; 10 \times 500 = 5000; 5000/45 = 111.11; 111.11$ mL of D50%

$35/45 = x/500; 35 \times 500 = 17{,}500; 17{,}500/45 = 388.89; 388.89$ mL of D5%

16.

50		15 parts of 50%
	20	
5		30 parts of 5%

$15 + 30 = 45$ parts total

$15/45 = x/300; 15 \times 300 = 4500; 4500/45 = 100; 100$ mL of Liposyn 50%

$30/45 = x/300; 30 \times 300 = 9000; 9000/45 = 200; 200$ mL of Liposyn 5%

17.

50		28 parts of 50%
	30	
2		20 parts of 2%

$28 + 20 = 48$ parts total

$28/48 = x/60; 28 \times 60 = 1680; 1680/48 = 35; 35$ g of 50%

$20/48 = x/60; 20 \times 60 = 1200; 1200/48 = 25; 25$ g of 2%

18.

70		20 parts of 70%
	60	
40		10 parts of 40%

$20 + 10 = 30$ parts total

$20/30 = x/1000; 20 \times 1000 = 20{,}000; 20{,}000/30 = 666.66$ mL of Travasol 70%

$10/30 = x/1000; 10 \times 1000 = 10{,}000; 10{,}000/30 = 333.33$ mL of Travasol 40%

19.

10		2 parts of 10%
	5	
3		5 parts of 3%

$2 + 5 = 7$ parts total

$2/7 = x/30; 2 \times 30 = 60; 60/7 = 8.57$ g of 10% bacitracin

$5/7 = x/30; 5 \times 30 = 150; 150/7 = 21.43$ g of 3% bacitracin

20. $30/454 = x/100; 30 \times 100 = 3000; 3000/454 = 6.61;$ the percentage strength is 6.61%.

21. $10\% = 10$ g/100g; 10 g/100 g $= x$ g/60 g; $10 \times 60 = 600$ g; $600/100 = 6; 6$ g of zinc in this compound

22. a. 5 g $\times 10 = 50$ g

b. 5 g

c. 7.5%

23. $8\% = 8$ g/100 g; $3\% = 3$ g/100 g $= x$ g/200 g; $3 \times 200 = 600; 600/100 = 6$ g

There are 8 g in 100 g.

There are 6 g in 200 g.

8 g $+ 6$ g $= 14$ g; 100 g $+ 200$ g $= 300$ g; 14 g$/300 = x/100; 14 \times 100 = 1400; 1400/300 = 4.666;$ the percentage strength is 4.67%.

24.

10		3.5 parts of 10%
	8.5	
5		1.5 parts of 5%

$3.5 + 1.5 = 5$ parts total

$3.5/5 = x/60; 3.5 \times 60 = 210; 210/5 = 42; 42$ g of 10% coal tar ointment

$1.5/5 = x/60; 1.5 \times 60 = 90; 90/5 = 18; 18$ g of 5% coal tar ointment

25. $70\% = 70$ mL/100 mL $= x$ mL/300 mL; $70 \times 300 = 21{,}000$; $21{,}000/100 = 210$

    210 mL of alcohol in 300 mL

    $95\% = 95$ mL/100 mL $= x$ mL/200 mL; $95 \times 200 = 19{,}000$; $19{,}000/100 = 190$;

    190 mL of alcohol in 200 mL

    $210 + 190 = 400$ mL of alcohol in 500 mL

    $400/500 = x/100$; $400 \times 100 = 40{,}000$; $40{,}000/500 = 80$

    The percentage strength is 80%.

26. $2000/70 = 28.57$; $28.57 \times 20 = 571.43$ mL of D70%

    $2000 - 571.43 = 1428.57$ mL of sterile water

27. $1000/70 = 14.29$; $14.29 \times 9 = 128.57$ mL of D70%

    $1000 - 128.57 = 871.43$ mL of sterile water

28. $500/50 = 10$; $10 \times 12 = 120$; 120 mL of D50%

    $500 - 120 = 380$ mL of sterile water

29. $600/50 = 12$; $12 \times 11 = 132$; 132 mL of D50%

    $600 - 132 = 468$ mL of sterile water

30. $350/5 = 70$; $70 \times 4 = 280$; 280 mL of D5%

    $350 - 280 = 70$ mL of sterile water

31. a. $1000/70 = 14.29$; $14.29 \times 16 = 228.57$ mL of D70%

    b. $1000/10 = 100$; $100 \times 4 = 400$; 400 mL of Aminosyn 10%

    c. $1000/20 = 50$; $50 \times 3 = 150$; 150 mL of Liposyn 20%

    d. 4 mEq/1 mL $= 15$ mEq/x mL; $1 \times 15 = 15$; $15/4 = 3.75$; 3.75 mL of NaCl

    e. 2 mEq/1 mL $= 30$ mEq/x mL; $1 \times 30 = 30$; $30/2 = 15$; 15 mL of KCl

    f. 3 mM/1 mL $= 10$ mM/x mL; $1 \times 10 = 10$; $10/3 = 3.33$; 3.33 mL of NaPhO$_4$

    g. 10 mL

    h. 100 units/1 mL $= 50$ units/x mL; $1 \times 50 = 50$; $50/100 = 0.5$; 0.5 mL of insulin

    i. $1000 - 811.15 = 188.85$ mL of sterile water (QSAD 100 mL)

    j. 1000 mL

Chapter 9

1. $\$126{,}000.00 + \$38{,}000.00 + \$12{,}000.00 + \$7{,}000.00 + \$1{,}500.00 + \$1{,}500.00 + \$2{,}500.00 + \$3{,}000.00 + \$425{,}000.00 = \$616{,}500.00$; $\$616{,}500.00 \times 0.25 = \$154{,}125.00$; $\$616{,}500 + \$154{,}125.00 = \$770{,}625.00$; the pharmacy income must be $\$770{,}625.00$ to meet the 25% goal

2. $\$1{,}401{,}750.00 - \$616{,}500.00 = \$785{,}250.00$; $\$785{,}250.00/\$1{,}401{,}750.00 \times 100$; $\$785{,}250.00/\$1{,}401{,}750.00 = 0.5602$; $0.5602 \times 100 = 56.02$, rounded to 56%; the pharmacy's current percentage profit is approximately 56%

3. a. $\$84.30 + \$5.24 = \$89.54$; $\$95.00 - \$89.54 = \$5.46$; the net profit is $\$5.46$

   b. $\$5.46/\$89.54 \times 100$; $\$5.46/\$89.54 = 0.061$; $0.061 \times 100 = 6.1$, rounded to 6; the percentage profit is approximately 6%

4. a. $\$32.50/500 = x/40$; $\$32.50 \times 40 = 1300$; $1300/500 = \$2.60$ for 40 tabs

      selling price $-$ overall costs $=$ net profit; $\$8.95 - \$2.60 - \$5.24 = \$1.11$

   b. markup $=$ selling price $-$ pharmacy's purchase price (for 40 tabs, not 500); $\$8.95 - \$2.60 = \$6.35$

      markup rate $=$ markup/pharmacy's purchase price; markup rate $= \$6.35/\$2.60 = \$2.44$; markup rate is 244%

5. $\$100.00 \times 5 = \$500.00$; $\$500.00 \times 0.15 = \$75.00$; $\$500.00 - \$75.00 = \$425.00$; the discounted price is $\$425.00$

6. $\$425.00 \times 0.2 = \$85.00$; $\$425.00 + \$85.00 = \$510.00$; $\$510.00/5 = \$102.00$; the selling price is $\$102$ per case; $\$102/24 = \$4.25$/tube

7. $\$0.28 - \$0.14 = \$0.14$; markup amount is $\$0.14$; $\$0.14/\$0.14 = 1$; $1 \times 100 = 100$; the markup is 100%

8. $\$2.15 - \$1.45 = \$0.70$; markup amount is $\$0.70$; $\$0.70/\$1.45 = 0.4828$; $0.4828 \times 100 = 48.28$, rounded to 48%; the markup is approximately 48%

9. $\$4.15 - \$3.25 = \$0.90$; markup amount is $\$0.90$; $\$0.90/\$3.25 = 0.2769$; $0.2769 \times 100 = 27.69$, rounded to 28; the markup is approximately 28%

10. $0.15 − $0.10 = $0.05; markup amount is $0.05; $0.05/$0.10 = 0.5; 0.5 × 100 = 50; the markup is 50%

11. $5.75 − $1.35 = $4.40; markup amount is $4.40; $4.40/1.35 = 3.259; 3.259 × 100 = 325.9, rounded to 326; the markup is approximately 326%

12. $14.95 − $8.50 = $6.45; markup amount is $6.45; $6.45/$8.50 = 0.7588; 0.7588 × 100 = 75.88, rounded to 76; the markup is approximately 76%

13. $94.45 × 0.12 = $11.33; $94.45 − $11.33 = $83.12; $83.12/120 = $0.6927; $0.6927 × 30 = $20.78; $20.78 + $4.50 = $25.28; the reimbursement amount is $25.28

14. $12.50 × 0.12 = $1.50; $12.50 − $1.50 = $11.00; $11.00/16 = $0.69; $0.69 × 4 = $2.76; the reimbursement amount is $2.76

15. $21.35 × 0.03 = $0.64; $21.35 + $0.64 = $21.99; $21.99 + $5.75 = $27.74; the reimbursement amount is $27.74

16. $90.32 × 0.03 = $2.71; $90.32 + $2.71 = $93.03; $93.03/480 = 0.1938; 0.1938 × 180 = $34.88;
$34.92 + $5.75 = $40.63; the reimbursement amount is $40.63

17. $62.00 × 0.02 = $1.24; $62.00 + $1.24 = $63.24; $63.24 + $1.50 = $64.74; $64.74 − $62.00 = $2.74; Khan's Pharmacy will make a profit of $2.74

$62.00 × .10 = $6.20; $62.00 − $6.20 = $55.80; $62.00 × 0.02 = $1.24; $62.00 + $1.24 = $63.24; $63.24 + $1.50 = $64.74; $64.74 − $55.80 = $8.94; Albright's Pharmacy will make a profit of $8.94

18. $18.75 × 0.10 = $1.88; $18.75 − $1.88 = $16.87; $16.87 + $6.00 = $22.87; $22.87 − $4.00 = $18.87; the pharmacy will make a profit of $18.87

19. a. $195.00 × 17 = $3315.00; $3315.00 + $60.00 = $3375.00; the HMO will reimburse $3375.00 for the month
    b. The pharmacy's drug costs were $867.50.
    c. The pharmacy made a profit.
    d. $3375.00 − $867.50 = $2507.50; the pharmacy made a profit of $2507.50

20. a. $120.00 × 46 = $5520.00; $5520.00 + $128.00 = $5648.00; the HMO will reimburse the pharmacy $5648.00
    b. The pharmacy's drug costs were $6187.50.
    c. The pharmacy lost money.
    d. $6187.50 − $5648.00 = $539.50; the pharmacy took a loss of $539.50

21. two bottles of 60

22. one bottle of 100

23. one bottle of 1000

24. zero

25. $188,737.50/$125,825.00 = 1.5; the turnover rate is 1.5

26. $546,210.00/$114,900.00 = 4.75; the turnover rate is 4.75

27. $18,452.00 − $12,208.00 = $6244.00; $6244.00/3 = $2081.33; the annual depreciation is $2081.33

28. $1478.00 − $850.00 = $628.00; $628.00/8 = $78.50; the annual depreciation is $78.50

Additional Assessments

Chapter 1 Quiz

Version A

1. Circle the fraction with the highest value.

   ¹⁄₁₀   ¹⁄₁₀₀   ¹⁄₁₀₀₀

2. Circle the fraction with the lowest value.

   ¹⁄₅   ³⁄₅   ⁵⁄₅

3. Reduce the following fraction to its lowest form.

   ⁹⁄₄₅

4. Express the following fraction as a decimal.

   ³⁄₈

5. Add the following fractions.

   2¹⁄₄ + ⁵⁄₆

6. Subtract the following fractions.

   4¹⁄₈ − ³⁄₄

7. Round the following number to the hundredths place.

   12.155012

8. Write the equivalent Arabic number for the following Roman numeral.

   MCDXCII

9. Write the equivalent Roman numeral for the following Arabic number.

   43

10. Rewrite the following number without using scientific notation.

    6.314×10^5

11. Rewrite the following number using scientific notation.

    0.000103

12. Add the following decimals.

    1.072 + 19.01 + 0.34 + 1.021

13. Subtract the following decimals.

    14.01 − 3.2 − 0.78

14. Multiply the following decimals.

    1.23 × 4.07

15. Divide the following decimals and round to the hundredths place.

    14/4.3

16. A student gets 22 questions correct on a 25-question pharmacy calculations exam. What is this grade expressed as a decimal? As a percentage?

17. A medication is to be given at 6:30 p.m. Express this time using 24-hour (military) time.

18. Convert the following 24-hour time to standard time, indicating a.m. or p.m.

    0058

19. You need to package 480 mL of cough syrup into 32 unit doses. How many milliliters will each individual dose contain?

20. Use the prescription below to answer the following questions.

    Note: The abbreviation *p.o.* means "by mouth," and the abbreviation *qam* means "every morning."

     Strattera 18 mg tabs

    Sig: 1 tab p.o. qam
    Disp: LX tablets

a. How many milligrams is the patient taking per dose?

b. How many tablets are to be dispensed?

c. How long will this prescription last?

Chapter 1 Quiz

Version B

1. Circle the fraction with the highest value.

   $7/12$ $3/12$ $5/12$

2. Circle the fraction with the lowest value.

   $7/13$ $7/8$ $7/1$

3. Circle the decimal with the highest value.

   2.097   0.9994   2.10003

4. Identify the number of significant figures for the following numbers, assuming that final zeros are not significant.

   a. 0.35 L

   b. 13.245 mcg

   c. 2.005 grains

   d. 423.220 mg

5. Round the following numbers to the hundredths place.

   a. 1.2459 g

   b. 0.04564 mL

   c. 124.809 L

   d. 1.005001 mcg

6. Express the following fraction as a decimal.

   $3/4$

7. Reduce the following fraction to its lowest form.

   $9/51$

8. Write the equivalent Roman numeral for the following Arabic number.

   404

9. Write the equivalent Arabic number for the following Roman numeral.

   MLXXII

10. Rewrite the following number using scientific notation.

    521,000

11. Rewrite the following number without using scientific notation.

    1.856×10^{-5}

12. Add the following fractions.

    $1\frac{2}{5} + 3\frac{2}{3}$

13. Subtract the following fractions.

    $2\frac{1}{4} - \frac{5}{12}$

14. Multiply the following decimals.

    2.3×10.1

15. Divide the following decimals.

    12/0.01

16. A student answers 24 questions correctly on a 40-question anatomy test. What is this grade expressed as a decimal? As a percentage?

17. A pharmacy technician signs for a shipment of antihistamines at 1330. What is this time expressed in standard time? Please indicate a.m. or p.m. in your answer.

18. Express 11:54 pm in 24-hour (military) time.

19. A patient takes 5 mL of morphine every six hours for pain control. How many milliliters will this patient use in seven days?

20. Use the prescription below to answer the following questions.

    Note: The abbreviation *p.o.* means "by mouth" and the abbreviation *qam* means "every morning."

    > ℞ **Apriso 3.75 g capsules**
    >
    > Sig: 1 capsule p.o. qam
    > Disp: XC

    a. How many capsules are to be dispensed?

    b. How long will this prescription last?

    c. How many grams of drug does the patient take each week?

Chapter 2 Quiz

Version A

1. Express the following ratios as fractions and reduce to their lowest terms, if applicable.

    a. 16:32

    b. 64:100

    c. 5:2

2. Reduce the following fractions to their lowest terms, and express them as ratios.

    a. ⁶⁄₈

    b. ⁸⁄₁₀

    c. ¹¹⁄₂

3. A 1:400 solution contains _____ g of active ingredient in _____ mL of total solution volume. Therefore, 800 mL of the same strength solution will contain _____ g of active ingredient.

4. What is the ratio, in lowest form, for a 5 mL dose of oral drug solution that contains 100 mg of morphine sulfate? Express your answer in milligrams:milliliter (mg:mL).

5. What is the ratio for 20 mg of lidocaine in 1 mL of solution for injection? Express your answer in milligrams:milliliter (mg:mL).

6. If 60 mg of Prozac is contained in three capsules, what is the ratio of milligrams of drug per capsule? Express your answer in lowest terms.

7. Convert the following fractions to percents, rounding to the nearest percent, if applicable.

    a. ⁴⁄₅

    b. ¹⁄₁

    c. ⁴⁄₆

    d. 2½

8. Convert the following percents to fractions. Reduce the fractions to their lowest terms.

    a. 19%

    b. 22%

    c. 125%

9. Convert the following percents to decimals.

    a. 73%

    b. 200%

    c. 0.1%

10. Convert the following percents to ratios, reducing where applicable.

    a. 44%

    b. 98%

    c. 130%

11. Solve for x in the following ratios. If applicable, round your answers to the nearest hundredth.

    a. $125/5 = 400/x$

    b. $66/88 = 3/x$

    c. $23/24 = 55/x$

    d. $x/120 = 14/15$

12. Convert the following volumes from liters (L) to milliliters (mL).

    $1 L = 1000 mL$

    a. 12 L = _____ mL

    b. 0.2 L = _____ mL

    c. 24.35 L = _____ mL

    d. 0.0145 L = _____ mL

13. If 1 grain of medication equals 60 mg, how many milligrams are in ¼ of a grain?

14. What is the percentage of error if the desired weight is 25 mcg and the measured weight is 24.1 mcg? Round your answer to the hundredths place.

15. What is the percentage of error if the desired weight is 375 mcg and the measured weight is 400 mcg? Round your answer to the hundredths place.

16. What is the percentage of error if the desired volume is 200 mL and the measured volume is 176 mL? Round your answer to the hundredths place.

17. You are working as a pharmacy technician in a hospital, measuring out the components for a TPN solution. You are instructed to measure 10 mL of multivitamin solution but discover that your measured volume was 9.79 mL. You are held to a standard of no more than 2% error. With that in mind, is your measurement within the permissible margin of error?

18. A prescriber ordered 125 mg of a drug. You have 25 mg strength tablets available. How many tablets will you need to fill the order?

19. Furosemide for injection comes in a concentration of 20 mg/2 mL. If you need to draw up 30 mg of this drug into a syringe, how many milliliters are required?

20. How many milliliters are required to deliver 375 mg of an oral solution of a drug that comes in a strength of 125 mg/5 mL?

Chapter 2 Quiz

Version B

1. Reduce the following fractions to their lowest terms, and express them as ratios.

    a. $^{14}/_{20}$

    b. $^{18}/_{50}$

    c. $^{10}/_{4}$

2. Express the following ratios as fractions and reduce the fractions to their lowest terms, if applicable.

    a. 24:30

    b. 100:8

    c. 17:4

3. A 3:10,000 solution contains _____ g of active ingredient in _____ mL of total solution volume. Therefore, 5,000 mL of the same strength solution will contain _____ g of active ingredient.

4. What is the ratio, in lowest form, for a drug solution that contains 375 mg of active drug in 5 mL of oral solution? Express your answer in milligrams:milliliter (mg:mL).

5. What is the ratio, in lowest form, for 975 mg of drug in three tablets?

6. Express the following fractions as percents, rounding to the nearest tenth of a percent, if applicable.

    a. $^{11}/_{12}$

    b. $^{25}/_{20}$

    c. $^{7}/_{9}$

7. Convert the following percents to decimals, rounding to the nearest hundredth of a percent, if applicable.

    a. 92½%

    b. 12.5%

    c. 105%

8. Convert the following percents to ratios, reducing where applicable.

    a. 22%

    b. 150%

    c. 0.50%

For questions 9–13, set up proportions to solve. Round your answers to the hundredths place, if applicable.

9. 54 is what percent of 500?

10. 45% of what number is 250?

11. What is 110% of 79?

12. What is 0.9% of 1200?

13. 13% of what number is 88?

14. Solve for x in the following ratios. If applicable, round your answers to the nearest hundredth.

    a. $4/5 = 40/x$

    b. $7/8 = x/12$

    c. $77/140 = 22/x$

    d. $132/400 = x/25$

15. Change the following volumes using the conversion of 1 fl oz = 30 mL. Round your answers to the tenths place, if applicable.

    a. 45 mL = _____ fl oz

    b. 135 mL = _____ fl oz

    c. 0.75 fl oz = _____ mL

    d. 1.45 fl oz = _____ mL

16. If there are 5 mL in 1 tsp, how many milliliters of medication does a patient ingest if she is instructed to take 2½ tsp of cough medicine per dose?

17. What is the percentage of error if the desired weight is 4500 mcg and the measured weight is 4532 mcg? Round your answer to the hundredths place.

18. What is the percentage of error if the desired volume is 100 mL and the measured volume is 972 mL? Round your answer to the hundredths place.

19. You are instructed to measure 45 mL of solution but discover that your measured amount is 43.5 mL. You are held to a standard of no greater than 4%. With that in mind, have you complied with this standard?

20. How many milliliters of injectable medication must you draw up if the order calls for 70 mg, and the concentration of the drug is 20 mg/mL?

Chapter 3 Quiz

Version A

1. Is this a valid DEA number for Dr. Harold Miller?

   AM 0535661

2. Is this a valid DEA number for Dr. Elizabeth Perkins-Ross?

   AP 6214023

3. Is this a valid DEA number for Dr. William B. Brooks?

   WB 0125820

4. Is this a valid DEA number for Steven Cooper, an advanced nurse practitioner?

   MC 5381022

5. Is this a valid DEA number for Dr. Francis Xavier, an oral surgeon?

   BX 1614230

6. How much medication should be dispensed for the following prescription?

    Ampicillin 250 mg capsules

   Sig: 1 tab po qid × 10 days

7. How much medication should be dispensed for the following prescription?

    Prednisone 5 mg tablets

   Sig: 1 tab po qid × 1 day
   then 1 tab po tid × 2 days
   then 1 tab po bid × 3 days
   then 1 tab po qd × 3 days

8. If a prescription calls for a patient to take 10 mL by mouth, twice daily for one week, how much medication will be dispensed?

9. How would 2% lidocaine for injection be expressed in milligrams/milliliter (mg/mL)? Reduce the amount to its lowest form.

10. If a patient is prescribed 240 mL of an oral solution that is dosed at 5 mL tid, how many full weeks will this medication last?

11. What is the days' supply for 90 capsules taken on a qid basis?

12. What is the days' supply for 120 tablets taken on a q12h basis?

13. If a patient has a prescription that requires two capsules to be taken each morning and one capsule to be taken each evening, how many days will 90 capsules last?

Write out the meanings of the following abbreviations.

14. mcg

15. tid

16. ac

17. AU

18. stat

19. pc

20. NKDA

Chapter 3 Quiz

Version B

1. Is this a valid DEA number for Dr. H. Patel?

   AP 7146587

2. Is this a valid DEA number for Dr. Patrick S. Chan?

   BC 3111414

3. Is this a valid DEA number for Clarice Bell, an advanced nurse practitioner?

   MA 4010322

4. Is this a valid DEA number for Dr. Wilford Rutherford?

   WR 2138512

5. Is this a valid DEA number for Dr. Jan Jankowski?

   AJ 05123657

6. How much medication should be dispensed for the following prescription?

    Nitroglycerin Sublingual Tablets

   Sig: 1 tab SL q4h prn chest pain

   Disp: LX

7. How much medication should be dispensed for the following prescription?

    Milk of Magnesia

   Sig: 5 mL po qid

   Disp: 2 weeks

8. If a patient is given a three-day prescription for a pain medication with the instructions below, what is the maximum number of tablets that can be taken?

   Sig: 1–2 tabs po q4–6h prn pain

   Disp: 3 days' supply

9. What is the days' supply for the following prescription?

    Diuretic

   Sig: 1 tablet po bid

   Disp: XL

10. What directions would you place on a patient's prescription label based on the directions below?

    2 gtts AU qid prn itching

11. What directions would you place on a patient's prescription label based on the directions below?

    1 tablet po tid ac

12. What directions would you place on a patient's prescription label based on the directions below?

    3 gtts OS q4h while awake × 3 days

13. What directions would you place on a patient's prescription label based on the directions below?

    1–2 capsules po q6h prn dizziness

Write out the meanings of the following abbreviations.

14. npo

15. gr

16. DAW

17. q8h

18. ud

19. D/C

20. OU

Chapter 4 Quiz

Version A

1. Change 3200 mg to grams by moving the decimal point.

2. Change 2.5 mg to micrograms by moving the decimal point.

Convert the following units using the ratio-proportion method. Round your answers to the nearest hundredth.

3. 650 mg = _____ mcg

4. 2.5 L = _____ mL

Convert the following units using the dimensional analysis method. Round your answers to the nearest hundredth.

5. 425 mg = _____ g

6. 3250 mL = _____ L

For questions 7–10, use the label provided below to determine the amount of drug that must be drawn up for the prescribed dose. Round your answers to the nearest hundredth.

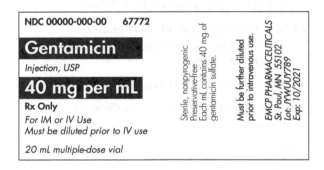

7. A prescriber has ordered 120 mg of gentamicin to be administered intramuscularly. How much gentamicin must be drawn up for this dose?

8. A prescriber has ordered 200 mg of gentamicin in 100 mL D$_5$W IVPB q8h. How much gentamicin must be drawn up for a single dose?

9. A prescriber has ordered 2 mg/kg of gentamicin q12h for a child who weighs 40 lb. How many milligrams of gentamicin will be needed for one dose?

10. Based on your answer for question 9, how much gentamicin must be drawn up for one dose?

Use the label provided below to determine the answers to questions 11–14. Round your answers to the nearest hundredth.

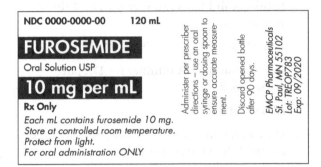

11. A patient is prescribed 6 mL of furosemide. How many milligrams is this?

12. A patient is prescribed 20 mg of furosemide. How many milliliters is this?

13. A patient is prescribed a furosemide dose of 40 mg po tid. How many milliliters will be required for one dose?

14. Based on what you calculated in question 13, how many milligrams will be administered each day?

15. A dose of Maalox is 30 mL. How many doses can be prepared from a 360 mL bottle?

16. A 12-year-old child weighs 80 lb and is to take acyclovir with a normal adult dose of 250 mg. Using Young's Rule, what is the appropriate pediatric dose for this child?

17. Using Clark's Rule, what is the appropriate pediatric dose for the child in question 16?

18. You have 1 pt of a solution that contains 8 g of active ingredient. How many milligrams of active ingredient are there in 5 mL of the solution? Round your answer to the nearest hundredth.

19. A patient is to receive 8 mg of haloperidol. The pharmacy has on hand a vial with a concentration of 10 mg/2 mL. How many milliliters will be needed to fill the prescription?

20. A patient is to receive 25,000 units of heparin in 500 mL of D₅W at a rate of 20 mL/hr. The pharmacy carries a stock solution of heparin with a concentration of 10,000 units/mL. How much heparin must be drawn up to prepare the IV solution?

Chapter 4 Quiz

Version B

1. Change 4800 mg to grams by moving the decimal point.

2. Change 5.2 mg to micrograms by moving the decimal point.

Convert the following units using the ratio-proportion method. Round your answers to the nearest hundredth.

3. 325 mg = _____ mcg

4. 4.5 L = _____ mL

Convert the following units using the dimensional analysis method. Round your answers to the nearest hundredth.

5. 155 mg = _____ g

6. 6250 mL = _____ L

For questions 7–10, use the label provided below to determine the amount of drug that must be drawn up to provide the prescribed dose. Round your answers to the nearest hundredth.

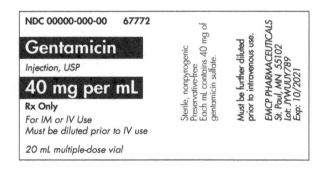

7. A prescriber has ordered 120 mg of gentamicin to be administered intramuscularly. How much gentamicin must be drawn up for this dose?

8. A prescriber has ordered 250 mg of gentamicin in 250 mL NS IVPB q12h. How much gentamicin must be drawn up for a single dose?

9. A prescriber has ordered 3 mg/kg of gentamicin q12h for a child who weighs 60 lb. How many milligrams of gentamicin will be needed for one dose?

10. Based on your answer for question 9, how much gentamicin must be drawn up for one dose?

Use the label provided below to determine the answers to questions 11–14. Round your answers to the nearest hundredth.

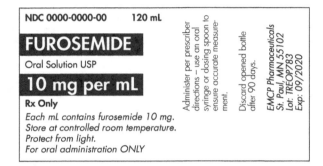

11. A patient is prescribed 5 mL of furosemide. How many milligrams is this?

12. A patient is prescribed 30 mg of furosemide. How many milliliters is this?

13. A patient is prescribed a furosemide dose of 20 mg po tid. How many milliliters will be required for one dose?

14. Based on what you calculated in question 13, how many milligrams will be administered each day?

15. A dose of Maalox is 30 mL. How many doses can be prepared from a 480 mL bottle?

16. A 6-year-old child weighs 40 lb and is to take acyclovir with a normal adult dose of 250 mg. Using Young's Rule, what is the appropriate pediatric dose for this child?

17. Using Clark's Rule, what is the appropriate pediatric dose for the child in question 16?

18. You have 1 pt of a solution that contains 8 g of active ingredient. How many milligrams of active ingredient are there in 30 mL of the solution? Round your answer to the nearest hundredth.

19. A patient is to receive 6 mg of haloperidol. The pharmacy has on hand a vial with a concentration of 10 mg/2 mL. How many milliliters will be needed to fill the prescription?

20. A patient is to receive 25,000 units of heparin in 500 mL of NS at a rate of 25 mL/hr. The pharmacy carries a stock solution of heparin with a concentration of 20,000 units/mL. How much heparin must be drawn up to prepare the IV solution?

Chapter 5 Quiz

Version A

1. Each tablespoon of liquid contains 250 mg of active ingredient. How many milligrams of active ingredient are contained in 1 pt?

Use the label provided below to determine the answers for questions 2–4.

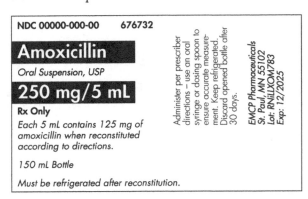

2. A pharmacy receives a prescription for amoxicillin 500 mg tid for 10 days. Based on the label provided above, how much will the patient need for a single dose?

3. Based on the label provided above, how many milligrams will the patient receive in one day?

4. Based on the label provided above, how many milligrams will the patient receive for the entire 10-day dosing regimen?

Convert the following temperatures from Celsius to Fahrenheit.

5. 42 °C

6. 70 °C

Convert the following temperatures from Fahrenheit to Celsius.

7. 98.6 °F

8. 32 °F

Use the label provided below to determine the answers for questions 9 and 10.

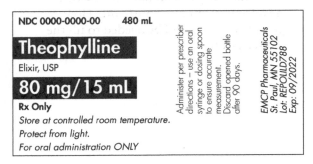

9. A prescriber has ordered 100 mg of theophylline elixir q6h. Based on the label provided above, how many milliliters are needed for one dose?

10. Based on the label provided above, how many milligrams will the patient receive in one day for this prescription?

Convert the following from pounds to kilograms. Round your answers to the nearest hundredth.

11. 150 lb

12. 75 lb

13. 200 lb

Convert the following from kilograms to pounds.

14. 25 kg

15. 38 kg

16. 80 kg

Use the label provided below to determine the answers for questions 17–20.

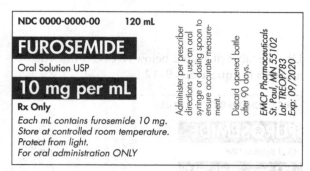

NDC 0000-0000-00   120 mL

FUROSEMIDE

Oral Solution USP

10 mg per mL

Rx Only

Each mL contains furosemide 10 mg.
Store at controlled room temperature.
Protect from light.
For oral administration ONLY

Administer per prescriber directions – use an oral syringe or dosing spoon to ensure accurate measurement.

Discard opened bottle after 90 days.

EMCP Pharmaceuticals
St. Paul, MN 55102
Lot: TREOP783
Exp: 09/2020

17. A prescriber has ordered a patient to receive ½ tsp bid for 14 days. How many milliliters will the patient receive per dose?

18. Based on the information provided in question 17, how many milliliters will the patient receive per day?

19. Based on the information provided in question 18, how many milliliters will the patient receive over the entire 14-day course of treatment?

20. Based on the information provided in question 19, how many milligrams will the patient receive over the entire 14-day course of treatment?

Chapter 5 Quiz

Version B

1. Each tablespoon of liquid contains 250 mg of active ingredient. How many milligrams of active ingredient are contained in 1 cup?

Use the label provided below to determine the answers for questions 2–4.

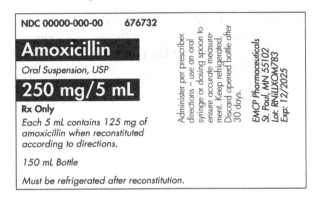

2. A pharmacy receives a prescription for amoxicillin 125 mg tid for 10 days. Based on the label provided above, how much will the patient need for a single dose?

3. Based on the label provided above, how many milligrams will the patient receive in one day?

4. Based on the label provided above, how many milligrams will the patient receive for the entire 10-day dosing regimen?

Convert the following temperatures from Celsius to Fahrenheit.

5. 54 °C

6. 72 °C

Convert the following temperatures from Fahrenheit to Celsius. Round your answers to the nearest hundredth.

7. 100 °F

8. 68 °F

Use the label provided below to determine the answers for questions 9–12.

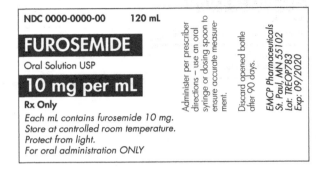

9. A prescriber has ordered a patient to receive ½ tsp bid for 14 days. How many milliliters will the patient receive per dose?

10. Based on the information provided in question 9, how many milliliters will the patient receive per day?

11. Based on the information provided in question 10, how many milliliters will the patient receive over the entire 14-day course of treatment?

12. Based on the information provided in question 11, how many milligrams will the patient receive over the entire 14-day course of treatment?

Use the label provided below to determine the answers to questions 13 and 14.

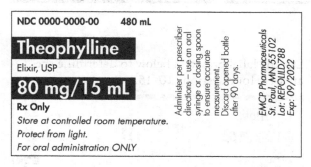

NDC 0000-0000-00	480 mL

Theophylline

Elixir, USP

80 mg/15 mL

Rx Only

Store at controlled room temperature.
Protect from light.
For oral administration ONLY

Administer per prescriber directions – use an oral syringe or dosing spoon to ensure accurate measurement. Discard opened bottle after 90 days.

EMCP Pharmaceuticals
St. Paul, MN 55102
Lot: REPOIILD788
Exp: 09/2022

13. A prescriber has ordered 100 mg of theophylline elixir q6h. Based on the label provided above, how many milliliters are needed for one dose?

14. Based on the adjacent label, how many milligrams will the patient receive in one day for this prescription?

Convert the following from pounds to kilograms. Round your answers to the nearest hundredth.

15. 155 lb

16. 70 lb

17. 210 lb

Convert the following from kilograms to pounds.

18. 20 kg

19. 36 kg

20. 81 kg

Chapter 6 Quiz

Version A

1. If a drug has a concentration of 50 mg/mL, how many milliliters are needed to prepare a 150 mg dose?

2. How many milliliters of a 1 g/5 mL solution must be drawn up for a 750 mg dose?

3. How many milligrams are contained in 50 mL of a 10 mg/mL solution?

4. How many milligrams are contained in 100 mL of a 1 g/10 mL solution?

Use the label provided below to determine the answers for questions 5–7.

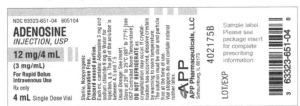

Images used with permission from Fresenius Kabi USA, LLC

5. The medication order calls for adenosine 10 mg in 50 mL NS to be administered IVPB over 20 min. What is the concentration of the IVPB in milligrams/milliliter (mg/mL)?

6. If the IVPB described in question 5 is administered three times in a 48-hour period, what is the total number of milligrams of adenosine that will be received by the patient?

7. If the IVPB described in question 5 is administered three times in a 48-hour period, what is the total number of milliliters of NS that will be received by the patient?

8. How many grams of drug are contained in 1000 mL of a 1:100 solution?

9. How many milliliters of a 1:5000 solution are required to provide 250 mg of drug?

Use the label provided below to determine the answers for questions 10–15.

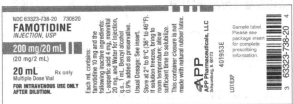

Images used with permission from Fresenius Kabi USA, LLC

10. A prescriber has ordered famotidine 40 mg in 50 mL D_5W to be administered over 15 min IVPB q8h. Based on the concentration from the vial label above, how many milliliters will be needed for this dose?

11. Based on the information provided in question 10, how many milliliters of famotidine will be required to prepare enough doses for a 24-hour period?

12. Based on the information provided above, how many milligrams of famotidine will be administered in a 24-hour period?

13. Based on the information provided above, how many milliliters of fluid will the patient receive from the IVPB in a 24-hour period?

14. Based on the information provided above, what is the concentration of the compounded IVPB in milligrams/milliliter (mg/mL)?

15. If the famotidine IVPB described above is administered to the patient for five days, how many total milligrams will the patient receive?

Use the label provided below to determine the answers for questions 16–18.

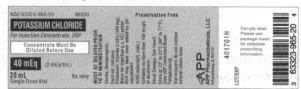

Images used with permission from Fresenius Kabi USA, LLC

16. A prescriber has ordered 1 L of D_5NS w/20 mEq of potassium chloride to run at 125 mL/hr. Based on the label provided above, how many milliequivalents (mEq) of potassium chloride will need to be drawn up for this dose?

17. Once the compounded sterile preparation (CSP) is prepared, what will the final concentration of the IV bag be in milliequivalents/milliliter (mEq/mL)?

18. If the IV solution runs continuously for 24 hr, infusing a total of 3 L of fluid, what is the total number of milliequivalents (mEq) that will be administered to the patient?

19. A patient is to receive 25,000 units of heparin in NS 500 mL continuous infusion. The pharmacy carries heparin with a concentration of 10,000 units/mL. How many milliliters of heparin will be needed to prepare the heparin infusion?

20. A patient is to receive 10 units of regular insulin subcutaneously every morning and 15 units of insulin every evening. The pharmacy carries regular insulin with a concentration of 100 units/mL. How many milliliters of regular insulin will the patient use in one day?

Chapter 6 Quiz

Version B

1. If a drug has a concentration of 50 mg/mL, how many milliliters are needed to prepare a 150 mg dose?

Use the label provided below to determine the answers for questions 2–4.

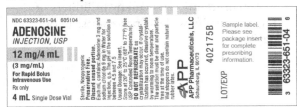

Images used with permission from Fresenius Kabi USA, LLC

2. The medication order calls for adenosine 10 mg in 50 mL NS to be administered IVPB over 20 min. What is the concentration of the IVPB in milligrams/milliliter (mg/mL)?

3. If the IVPB described in question 2 is administered three times in a 48-hour period, what is the total number of milligrams of adenosine that will be received by the patient?

4. If the IVPB described above is administered three times in a 48-hour period, what is the total number of milliliters of NS that will be received by the patient?

5. How many milliliters of a 1 g/10 mL solution must be drawn up for a 750 mg dose?

6. How many milligrams are contained in 50 mL of a 100 mg/mL solution?

7. How many milligrams are contained in 250 mL of a 1 g/10 mL solution?

8. How many grams of drug are contained in 500 mL of a 1:100 solution?

9. How many milliliters of a 1:5000 solution are required to provide 750 mg of drug?

Use the label provided below to determine the answers to questions 10–15.

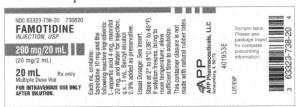

Images used with permission from Fresenius Kabi USA, LLC

10. A prescriber has ordered famotidine 20 mg in 50 mL D$_5$W to be administered over 15 min IVPB q8h. Based on the concentration from the vial label above, how many milliliters will be needed for this dose?

11. Based on the information provided in question 10, how many milliliters of famotidine will be required to prepare enough doses for a 24-hour period?

12. Based on the information provided above, how many milligrams of famotidine will be administered in a 24-hour period?

13. Based on the information provided above, how many milliliters of fluid will the patient receive from the IVPB in a 24-hour period?

14. Based on the information provided above, what is the concentration of the compounded IVPB in milligrams/milliliter (mg/mL)?

15. If the famotidine IVPB described above is administered to the patient for five days, how many total milligrams will the patient receive?

Use the label provided below to determine the answers to questions 16–18.

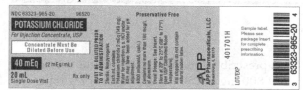

Images used with permission from Fresenius Kabi USA, LLC

16. A prescriber has ordered 1 L of D_5W w/30 mEq of potassium chloride to run at 125 mL/hr. Based on the label provided above, how many milliequivalents (mEq) of potassium chloride will need to be drawn up for this dose?

17. Once the compounded sterile preparation (CSP) is prepared, what will the final concentration of the IV bag be in milliequivalents/milliliter (mEq/mL)?

18. If the IV solution runs continuously for 24 hr, infusing a total of 3 L of fluid, what is the total number of milliequivalents (mEq) that will be administered to the patient?

19. A patient is to receive 25,000 units of heparin in NS 500 mL continuous infusion. The pharmacy carries heparin with a concentration of 20,000 units/mL. How many milliliters of heparin will be needed to prepare the heparin infusion?

20. A patient is to receive 10 units of regular insulin subcutaneously every morning, as well as 15 units after lunch, and 25 units every evening. The pharmacy carries regular insulin with a concentration of 100 units/mL. How many milliliters of regular insulin will the patient use in one day?

Chapter 7 Quiz

Version A

1. How many grams of dextrose are in 600 mL of D_5W?

2. How many grams of sodium chloride are in 250 mL of NS?

3. If there are 50 g of dextrose in a 500 mL IV bag, what is the percentage strength of the solution?

4. Use the label provided below to determine the percentage strength of the solution.

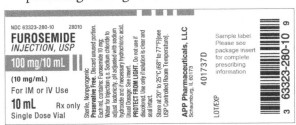

Images used with permission from Fresenius Kabi USA, LLC

5. Express the components of a 7% solution of dextrose in the form of a w/v solution.

6. A 1 L IV is administered at 75 mL/hr. How long will the IV bag last?

7. A prescriber has ordered D_5W ½NS 1000 mL to run at 100 mL/hr. How many bags will be needed in a 24-hour period?

8. A prescriber has ordered a 1 L IV bag to be infused over 24 hr. What is the IV flow rate in milliliters per hour (mL/hr)?

9. A physician has ordered a 100 mL IVPB with 500 mg of Solu-Cortef to be administered over 4 hr. What dose of the drug is being administered per hour?

10. An IV has a total volume of 500 mL and is being administered over 3 hr using microdrip tubing with a drop factor of 15 gtts/mL. What is the rate in drops per minute (gtts/min)?

11. An IV of NS 500 mL with 20,000 units of heparin is administered at a rate of 40 mL/hr using a drop factor of 20 gtts/mL. How many drops per minute (gtts/min) is that?

12. A prescriber has ordered a dopamine drip of 800 mg in 250 mL D_5W. The IV will be administered at 8 mL/hr through the tubing that has a drop factor of 15 gtts/mL. How many milligrams of dopamine are in each drop?

Use the medication order provided below to determine the answers to questions 13–17.

ID#: LM13691714			Memorial Hospital
Name: Gentry, Stephen			
DOB: 03/23/59			
Room: 733			
Dr: Melvin Scott, M.D.			Physician's Medication Order
ALLERGY OR SENSITIVITY		**DIAGNOSIS**	
PCN, latex		cardiac dysrhythmia	
DATE	TIME	ORDERS	PHYSICIAN'S SIG.
7/4/2018	3:24 p.m.	D5NS w/40 mEq KCl	
		@125 mL/hr	
			M. Scott, M.D.

13. How many grams of dextrose will the patient receive in each IV bag?

14. How many grams of dextrose will the patient receive in a 24-hour period?

15. How many grams of sodium chloride will the patient receive in each IV bag?

16. How many grams of sodium chloride will the patient receive in a 24-hour period?

17. How many milliequivalents (mEq) of KCl will the patient receive in a 24-hour period?

Use the IV label provided below to determine the answers to questions 18–20.

```
***Large-Volume Parenteral***
        Memorial Hospital
Name: Shelby Corvan        Room: 852
Pt. ID#: CØ433975          Rx#: 385226
_____

    Aminophylline 1 gram
    D₅W 250 mL
    Rate: 10 mL/hr

Expires _____
RPh _____
Tech _____

   Keep refrigerated—warm to room temperature
              before use.
```

18. How many grams of dextrose will the patient receive in a 24-hour period?

19. How many milligrams of aminophylline will the patient receive in a 24-hour period?

20. How many milliliters of fluid will the patient receive in a 24-hour period?

Chapter 7 Quiz

Version B

1. How many grams of sodium chloride are in 500 mL of NS?

2. How many grams of dextrose are in 700 mL of $D_{10}W$?

3. If there are 25 g of dextrose in a 500 mL IV bag, what is the percentage strength of the solution?

4. Use the label provided below to determine the percentage strength of the solution.

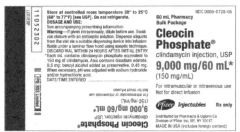

Copyright Pfizer Inc. Used with permission.

5. A prescriber has ordered D_5NS 1 L to run at 100 mL/hr. How many bags will be needed over a 24-hour period?

6. Express the components of a 15% solution of dextrose in the form of a w/v solution.

7. A 1 L IV is infused at 50 mL/hr. How long will the IV bag last?

8. A physician has ordered a 150 mL IVPB with a 500 mg solution of Solu-Cortef to be administered over 4 hr. What dose of the drug is being administered per hour?

9. A prescriber has ordered a 500 mL IV bag to be infused over 24 hr. What is the IV flow rate in milliliters per hour (mL/hr)?

10. An IV has a total volume of 250 mL and is being administered over 2 hr using macrodrip tubing with a drop factor of 15 gtts/mL. What is the rate in drops per minute?

11. An IV of NS 500 mL with 20,000 units of heparin is being administered at a rate of 40 mL/hr using macrodrip tubing with a drop factor of 20 gtts/mL. How many drops per minute (gtts/min) is that?

12. A prescriber has ordered a dopamine drip of 800 mg in 250 mL D_5W. The IV will be administered at 8 mL/hr through tubing that has a drop factor of 15 gtts/mL. How many milligrams of dopamine are in each drop?

Use the label provided below to determine the answers to questions 13–15.

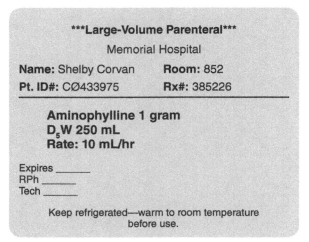

Large-Volume Parenteral

Memorial Hospital

Name: Shelby Corvan   **Room:** 852
Pt. ID#: CØ433975   **Rx#:** 385226

Aminophylline 1 gram
D_5W 250 mL
Rate: 10 mL/hr

Expires _____
RPh _____
Tech _____

Keep refrigerated—warm to room temperature before use.

13. How many grams of dextrose will the patient receive in a 24-hour period?

14. How many milligrams of aminophylline will the patient receive in a 24-hour period?

15. How many milliliters of fluid will the patient receive in a 24-hour period?

Use the medication order provided below to determine the answers for questions 16–20.

ID#: LM13691714			Memorial Hospital	
Name: Gentry, Stephen				
DOB: 03/23/59				
Room: 733			Physician's	
Dr: Melvin Scott, M.D.			Medication Order	
ALLERGY OR SENSITIVITY			DIAGNOSIS	
PCN, latex			cardiac dysrhythmia	
DATE	TIME	ORDERS		PHYSICIAN'S SIG.
7/4/2018	3:24 p.m.	D5NS w/40 mEq KCl		
		@125 mL/hr		
				M. Scott, M.D.

16. How many grams of dextrose will the patient receive in each IV bag?

17. How many grams of dextrose will the patient receive in a 24-hour period?

18. How many grams of sodium chloride will the patient receive in each IV bag?

19. How many grams of sodium chloride will the patient receive in a 24-hour period?

20. How many milliequivalents (mEq) of KCl will the patient receive in a 24-hour period?

Chapter 8 Quiz

Version A

Use the information provided below to answer questions 1 and 2.

Prepare an IV solution with a final concentration of 8% and a total volume of 500 mL. The pharmacy carries the dextrose stock solutions $D_{70}W$ and D_5W.

1. How many milliliters of $D_{70}W$ are needed to prepare the solution?

2. How many milliliters of D_5W are needed to prepare the solution?

Use the information provided below to answer questions 3–7.

Prepare 400 mL of $D_{15}W$ using $D_{70}W$ and D_5W.

3. How many parts of $D_{70}W$ will be needed to prepare the solution?

4. How many parts of D_5W will be needed to prepare the solution?

5. How many total parts are there in the solution?

6. How many milliliters of $D_{70}W$ are needed to prepare the solution?

7. How many milliliters of D_5W are needed to prepare the solution?

8. A pharmacy has received a prescription for 40 g of a 3% triamcinolone ointment. How many grams of triamcinolone will be needed to prepare the prescription?

9. Prepare a special dilution of gentamicin with a total volume of 5 mL and a concentration of 5 mg/mL. Use a stock solution of gentamicin 10 mg/mL and sterile water. What volume of gentamicin stock solution is needed to prepare this special dilution? What volume of sterile water is needed?

10. Prepare a prescription that mixes 10 g of acyclovir and 40 g of petrolatum. What is the percentage strength of the preparation?

For questions 11–20, use the TPN order provided below, along with the various stock solutions carried by your pharmacy, to determine the volume of each base solution and additive.

10/23/2019		
TPN Standing Orders		
Base Solution:	Dextrose 15%	
	Aminosyn 3%	
	Liposyn 3%	
	Sterile water QSAD to 1500 mL	
Additives:	Sodium chloride 40 mEq/L	
	Potassium chloride 20 mEq/L	
	Potassium phosphate 10 mM/L	
	Sodium phosphate 3 mM/L	
	Magnesium sulfate 10 mEq/L	
	MVI 10 mL	
Total volume:	1500 mL	
Flow rate:	60 mL/hr	
Physician:	Dr. Sharon Gennex	
	Signature: *Sharon Gennex, M.D.*	

Patient: Friedman, Fayth
Room #: TCU-14
DOB: 06/27/61
Allergies: NKDA
Pt. ID #: GKM00043657

The pharmacy carries the following stock solutions:

Dextrose 70%
Aminosyn 10%
Liposyn 20%
Sodium chloride 4 mEq/mL
Potassium chloride 2 mEq/mL
Potassium phosphate 3 mM/mL
Sodium phosphate 3 mM/mL
Magnesium sulfate 4.06 mEq/mL
MVI 10 mL

11. Dextrose

12. Aminosyn

13. Liposyn

14. Sodium chloride

15. Potassium chloride

16. Potassium phosphate

17. Sodium phosphate

18. Magnesium sulfate

19. MVI

20. Sterile water

Chapter 8 Quiz

Version B

Use the information below to answer questions 1 and 2.

You are to prepare an IV solution with a final concentration of 7.5% and a total volume of 1000 mL. The pharmacy carries the dextrose stock solutions $D_{70}W$ and D_5W. How much of each solution will you need to prepare the desired solution?

1. How much $D_{70}W$ is needed?

2. How much D_5W is needed?

Use the information provided to answer questions 3–7.

Prepare 700 mL of $D_{18}W$ using $D_{70}W$ and D_5W.

3. How many parts of $D_{70}W$ are needed?

4. How many parts of D_5W are needed?

5. How many total parts are there?

6. How many milliliters of $D_{70}W$ are needed?

7. How many milliliters of D_5W are needed?

8. A pharmacy received a prescription for 50 g of a 5% triamcinolone cream. How many grams of triamcinolone will be needed to prepare this prescription?

9. Prepare a prescription that mixes 8 g of acyclovir and 42 g of petrolatum. What is the percentage strength of the prescription?

10. Prepare a special dilution of Decadron with a total volume of 4 mL and a concentration of 1 mg/mL. Use a stock solution of Decadron 4 mg/mL and sterile water. What is the volume of the Decadron stock solution needed to prepare this special dilution? What is the volume of sterile water needed?

For questions 11–20, use the TPN order provided below, along with the various stock solutions carried by your pharmacy, to determine the volume of each base solution and additive.

10/23/2019		
TPN Standing Orders		Patient: Friedman, Fayth
Base Solution: Dextrose 12%		Room #: TCU-14
Aminosyn 5%		DOB: 06/27/61
Liposyn 2%		Allergies: NKDA
Sterile water QSAD to 1500 mL		Pt. ID #: GKM00043657
Additives: Sodium chloride 40 mEq/L		
Potassium chloride 20 mEq/L		
Potassium phosphate 10 mM/L		
Sodium phosphate 3 mM/L		
Magnesium sulfate 10 mEq/L		
MVI 10 mL		
Total volume: 1500 mL		
Flow rate: 80 mL/hr		
Physician: Dr. Sharon Gennex		
Signature: _Sharon Gennex, M.D._		

The pharmacy carries the following stock solutions:

Dextrose 70%
Aminosyn 10%
Liposyn 20%
Sodium chloride 4 mEq/mL
Potassium chloride 2 mEq/mL
Potassium phosphate 3 mM/mL
Sodium phosphate 3 mM/mL
Magnesium sulfate 4.06 mEq/mL

11. Dextrose

12. Aminosyn

13. Liposyn

14. Sodium chloride

15. Potassium chloride

16. Potassium phosphate

17. Sodium phosphate

18. Magnesium sulfate

19. MVI

20. Sterile water

Chapter 9 Quiz

Version A

Use the overhead expenses of Healthmart Pharmacy to answer questions 1–3.

pharmacist salary	$155,000.00
technician salary	$51,000.00
rent	$23,000.00
utilities	$6,000.00
computer maintenance	$4,000.00
software subscriptions	$2,000.00
liability insurance	$4,000.00
business insurance	$4,000.00
drug purchases	$750,000.00

1. If an 18% profit is desirable, what must the pharmacy's income be to meet this goal?

2. If the pharmacy's income is $1,401,489.00, what is its percentage profit?

3. If the pharmacy's income is $1,191,692.00, what is its percentage profit?

For questions 4–6 below, calculate the markup rate for the following prescription drug items. Round your answers to whole percents.

4. Medication: amoxicillin 250 mg
   Pharmacy's purchase price: $6.50
   Count: 100 capsules
   Amount dispensed: 30 capsules
   Pharmacy's selling price: $14.80

5. Medication: furosemide 40 mg
   Pharmacy's purchase price: $83.50
   Count: 500 tablets
   Amount dispensed: 100 tablets
   Pharmacy's selling price: $22.50

6. Medication: cyclobenzaprine 10 mg
   Pharmacy's purchase price: $4.36
   Count: 100 tablets
   Amount dispensed: 30 tablets
   Pharmacy's selling price: $5.25

7. Acetaminophen tablets regularly sell for $4.76. The medication is currently discounted at 40%. What is the discounted selling price of the acetaminophen tablets?

8. Cough syrup regularly sells for $5.19. The medication is currently discounted at 25%. What is the discounted selling price of the cough syrup?

9. The pharmacy purchase price of antiviral ointment is $12.00 per tube. The standard markup is 30%. Calculate the selling price of a case of 12 tubes.

Use the information below to answer questions 10–13.

PharMed HMO pays a per patient capitation fee of $275.00 per month to Healthy Pharmacy. Healthy Pharmacy contracts with PharMed HMO to serve 10 of Healthy Pharmacy's clients. Five of the PharMed HMO clients get prescriptions filled during the month of June; the other five patients do not get any prescriptions filled in June. The pharmacy's drug costs for these prescriptions are as follows:

Patient #1:	$89.63
Patient #2:	$126.54 (total cost for two prescriptions)
Patient #3:	$420.45 (total cost for five prescriptions)
Patient #4:	$117.50
Patient #5:	$46.75

10. What is the total amount that the HMO reimbursed the pharmacy for capitation fees?

11. What is the pharmacy's drug cost for all of the prescriptions on this plan?

12. Did the pharmacy make a profit or lose money?

13. If the pharmacy made a profit, what was the amount? If the pharmacy took a loss, what was the amount?

14. A pharmacy manager determines that the pharmacy's average inventory value is $176,000.00. The pharmacy's annual purchase amount is $585,000.00. What is the pharmacy's turnover rate?

15. The pharmacy's computer hardware costs $5,000.00. Its estimated useful life is five years, and the disposal value is $500.00. What is the annual depreciation?

16. The pharmacy purchased a 100 count bottle of azithromycin (Zithromax) 500 mg tablets at AWP plus 3%. The pharmacy charges a $5.00 dispensing fee for this prescription. If the AWP is $82.00 and the patient receives a prescription for six tablets, what is the amount that the pharmacy will submit for reimbursement?

For items 17–20, determine the number of units that need to be reordered for each item based on the current inventory and the number of units or packages needed to bring the item up to at least the minimum par level.

Drug	Count/ Package Size	Minimum Par Level	Maximum Par Level	Current Inventory	Reorder Amount
17. cefaclor 500 mg tab	100	250	500	140	
18. cefprozil 500 mg tab	50	30	100	34	
19. doxycycline 50 mg cap	50	30	200	100	
20. furosemide 40 mg tab	100	250	1000	107	

Chapter 9 Quiz

Version B

Use the overhead expenses of Gateway Pharmacy to answer questions 1–3.

pharmacist salaries	$278,000.00
technician salaries	$122,000.00
rent	$50,000.00
utilities	$6,000.00
computer maintenance	$4,000.00
software subscriptions	$2,000.00
liability insurance	$4,000.00
business insurance	$4,000.00
drug purchases	$1,115,000.00

1. If an 18% profit is desirable, what must the pharmacy's income be to meet this goal?

2. If the pharmacy's income is $2,401,489.00, what is its percentage profit?

3. If the pharmacy's income is $1,991,692.00, what is its percentage profit?

4. Acetaminophen tablets regularly sell for $4.76. The medication is currently discounted at 40%. What is the discounted selling price of the acetaminophen tablets?

5. Cough syrup regularly sells for $5.19. The medication is currently discounted at 25%. What is the discounted selling price of the cough syrup?

6. The pharmacy purchase price of antiviral ointment is $12.00 per tube. The standard markup is 30%. Calculate the selling price of a case of 12 tubes.

For questions 7–9 below, calculate the markup rate for the following prescription drug items. Round your answers to whole percents.

7. Medication: amoxicillin 250 mg
   Pharmacy's purchase price: $6.50
   Count: 100 capsules
   Amount dispensed: 30 capsules
   Pharmacy's selling price: $14.80

8. Medication: furosemide 40 mg
   Pharmacy's purchase price: $83.50
   Count: 500 tablets
   Amount dispensed: 100 tablets
   Pharmacy's selling price: $22.50

9. Medication: cyclobenzaprine 10 mg
   Pharmacy's purchase price: $4.36
   Count: 100 tablets
   Amount dispensed: 30 tablets
   Pharmacy's selling price: $5.25

Use the information below to answer questions 10–13.

Grand Rapids HMO pays a per patient capitation fee of $155.00 per month to City Pharmacy. City Pharmacy contracts with Grand Rapids HMO to serve 15 of City Pharmacy's clients. Seven of the Grand Rapids HMO clients get prescriptions filled during the month of June; the other eight patients do not get any prescriptions filled in June. The pharmacy's drug costs for these prescriptions are as follows:

Patient #1:	$89.63
Patient #2:	$126.54 (total cost for two prescriptions)
Patient #3:	$420.45 (total cost for five prescriptions)
Patient #4:	$117.50
Patient #5:	$46.75
Patient #6:	$27.23
Patient #7:	$34.87

10. What is the total amount that the HMO reimbursed the pharmacy for capitation fees?

11. What is the pharmacy's drug cost for all of the prescriptions on this plan?

12. Did the pharmacy make a profit or lose money?

13. If the pharmacy made a profit, what was the amount? If the pharmacy took a loss, what was the amount?

14. A pharmacy manager determines that the pharmacy's average inventory value is $228,050.00. The pharmacy's annual purchase amount is $725,000.00. What is the pharmacy's turnover rate?

15. The pharmacy's delivery van cost $15,000.00. Its estimated useful life is 10 years, and the disposal value is $1000.00. What is the annual depreciation?

16. The pharmacy purchased a 100 count bottle of furosemide 20 mg tablets at AWP plus 3%. The pharmacy charges a $5.00 dispensing fee on this prescription. If the AWP is $42.00 and the patient receives a prescription for 30 tablets, what is the amount that the pharmacy will submit for reimbursement?

For items 17–20, determine the number of units that need to be reordered for each item based on the current inventory and the number of units or packages needed to bring the item up to at least the minimum par level.

Drug	Count/Package Size	Minimum Par Level	Maximum Par Level	Current Inventory	Reorder Amount
17. metformin 500 mg tab	100	250	500	200	
18. citalopram 40 mg cap	100	150	300	130	
19. raloxifene 60 mg cap	50	30	200	100	
20. lisinopril 5 mg tab	100	250	500	260	

Additional Assessments Answer Keys

Chapter 1 Quiz

Version A

1. $\frac{1}{10}$

   Because the numerators are the same, you look at the denominators, and $\frac{1}{10}$ has the smallest denominator.

2. $\frac{1}{5}$

   Because the denominators are the same, you look at the numerators, and $\frac{1}{5}$ has the smallest numerator.

3. $\frac{1}{5}$

   Both the numerator and the denominator may be divided by 9.

4. 0.375

5. $3\frac{1}{12}$

   A common denominator of either 24 or 12 may be used to convert the fractions.

6. $3\frac{3}{8}$

   $4\frac{1}{8}$ is made into the improper fraction of $\frac{33}{8}$; $\frac{3}{4}$ is made into the equivalent fraction of $\frac{6}{8}$, which is subtracted to give $\frac{27}{8}$. This is converted to the mixed number of $3\frac{3}{8}$.

7. 12.16. Identify the 5 in the hundredths place. The number to the right of it is 5 or greater. Therefore, the 5 is rounded up to 6.

8. 1492

9. XLIII

10. 631400. The decimal point is moved three digits to the right to account for 3 of the 5 zeros. Then two more zeros are added to account for the last two.

11. 1.03×10^{-4}

    A decimal point is placed between the 1 and the 0; then four places are counted to the left.

12. 21.443

13. 10.03

14. 5.0061

15. 3.26

    The answer is 3.255, which is to the thousandths place. Identify the 5 in the hundredths place. The number to the right of it is 5 or greater. Therefore, the number is rounded up to 3.26.

16. 0.88 and 88%

    Divide 22 by 25 to get the decimal (0.88). Take the decimal (0.88) and multiply it by 100 to get the percentage (88%).

17. 1830

    Military, or 24-hour time, is based on the number of hours and minutes past midnight. It takes 12 hours to get to noon, and 6 more hours to get to 6:00 p.m. Add the minutes without a colon preceding it.

18. 12:58 a.m.

    The stated time has not passed a full hour after midnight; therefore, the first two digits are 00. Add a colon and then add the minutes. Signify the time as "a.m."

19. 15 mL

    Take the total amount (480 mL) and divide it by 32 doses. The answer is 15 mL/dose.

20. a. 18 mg

    b. 60 tablets

    c. 60 days or approximately 2 months

Chapter 1 Quiz

Version B

1. $\frac{7}{12}$

   All of the possible answers have the same denominators; therefore, the answer choice with the largest numerator will have the highest value.

2. $\frac{7}{13}$

   All of the possible answers have the same numerators; therefore, the answer choice with the largest denominator will have the lowest value.

3. 2.10003

The first and third choices have the number 2 in the highest place value (the ones place). That observation eliminates the middle choice as a possible answer. Then you must look at the next highest place value in the two remaining choices: One choice has a 0 and the other choice has a 1. The larger digit in that place value determines which number has the higher value. Therefore, the answer is 2.10003.

4. a. Two significant figures. Begin counting at the first nonzero digit.

   b. Five significant figures. All five digits are nonzero.

   c. Four significant figures. All zeros between nonzero digits are significant.

   d. Five significant figures. Trailing zeros are usually not significant unless the measurement recorded is known to be accurate to the level of the trailing zero(s).

5. a. 1.25 g

   b. 0.05 mL

   c. 124.81 L

   d. 1.01 mcg

6. 0.75

7. $3/17$

   Both the numerator and denominator may be divided by 3.

8. CDIV

9. 1072

10. 5.21×10^5

    Place the decimal so that it makes a number larger or equal to 1, yet less than 10. Then account for the decimal point shifts in the exponent.

11. 0.00001856

    Place the decimal so that it makes a number larger or equal to 1, yet less than 10. Then account for the decimal point shifts in the exponent.

12. $5\frac{1}{15}$

    Convert both mixed numbers to the improper fractions of $7/5$ and $11/3$. The common denominator of these improper fractions is 15. Multiply $7/5$ by $3/3$ to get $21/15$. Then, multiply $11/3$ by $5/5$ to get $55/15$. Add the numerators of these equivalent fractions to get $76/15$. Finally, convert to a mixed number by division to arrive at $5\frac{1}{15}$.

13. $1\frac{10}{12}$, reduced to $1\frac{5}{6}$

    Convert $2\frac{1}{4}$ to the improper fraction of $9/4$. Then find the common denominator of $9/4$ and $5/12$, which is 12. Multiply $9/4$ by $3/3$ to get $27/12$. Subtract the numerators to get $22/12$. Convert it to a mixed number by division to get $1\frac{10}{12}$, which can be reduced to $1\frac{5}{6}$.

14. 23.23

15. 1200

16. 0.6 and 60%

    Divide 24 by 40 to arrive at 0.6. Multiply 0.6 by 100 and add the percent sign.

17. 1:30 p.m.

18. 2354

    To convert to 24-hour time, you must consider how many hours past midnight have elapsed. It took 12 hours to get to noon, and 11 more hours to get to 11:00 p.m. After that is determined, add the minutes without a colon preceding it.

19. 140 mL

    A medication that is taken every 6 hours amounts to four doses per day. Four doses per day times 7 days equal 28 doses. Each dose is 5 mL; therefore, 140 mL of morphine are used by the patient.

20. a. 90 capsules

    b. 90 days or approximately three months, given a dosing schedule of one capsule per day

    c. 26.25 g

       3.75 g per dose times seven doses per week

Chapter 2 Quiz

Version A

1. a. ½

   b. ¹⁶⁄₂₅

   Reduce from ⁶⁴⁄₁₀₀.

   c. ⁵⁄₂

2. a. 3:4

   b. 4:5

   c. 3:2

   Convert ½ to the improper fraction of ³⁄₂.

3. 1; 400; 2

4. 20 mg:1 mL

   Reduce from 100 mg:5 mL.

5. 20 mg:1 mL

6. 20 mg:1 capsule

   Reduce from 60 mg:3 capsules by dividing both sides of the ratio by 3.

7. a. 80%

   b. 100%

   c. 67%

   d. 250%

   Convert 2½ to the improper fraction ⁵⁄₂, and then apply the standard rules.

8. a. ¹⁹⁄₁₀₀

   b. ¹¹⁄₅₀

   Reduce from ²²⁄₁₀₀.

   c. ⁵⁄₄

   Reduce from ¹²⁵⁄₁₀₀.

9. a. 0.73

   b. 2

   c. 0.001

10. a. 11:25

   Convert 44% to a fraction to yield ⁴⁴⁄₁₀₀; reduce to its lowest terms of ¹¹⁄₂₅.

   b. 49:50

   c. 13:10

11. a. $x = 16$

   Cross multiply $125x = 400 \times 5$; $125x = 2000$; $125x/125 = 2000/125$; $x = 16$.

   b. $x = 4$

   c. $x = 57.39$

   d. $x = 112$

12. a. 12,000 mL

   Using ratio-proportion, 1 L/1000 mL = 12 L/x mL

   b. 200 mL

   c. 24,350 mL

   d. 14.5 mL

13. 15 mg (60 mg $\times$ ¼ = 15 mg)

   You also may have your students draw a 60 mg pie or bar and divide it into 4 equal pieces.

14. 3.6%

   The applicable formula is amount of error/quantity desired $\times$ 100 = percentage of error. Therefore, (25 mcg − 24.1 mcg)/25 mcg $\times$ 100 = 0.9 mcg/25 mcg $\times$ 100, which yields a percentage of error of 3.6%.

15. 6.67%

   25 mcg/375 mcg $\times$ 100 = 6.67%

16. 12%

17. No. The percentage of error is 2.1%.

   (10 mL − 9.79 mL)/10 mL $\times$ 100 = 2.1%

18. 5 tablets

   Using the ratio-proportion method, 25 mg/1 tablet = 125 mg/x tablets

19. 3 mL

   20 mg/ 2 mL = 30 mg/x mL

20. 15 mL

   125 mg/5 mL = 375 mg/x mL

Chapter 2 Quiz

Version B

1. a. 7:10

   b. 9:25

   c. 5:2

2. a. 4/5

   b. 25/2

   c. 17/4

3. 3; 10,000; 1.5

4. 75 mg:1 mL

   Reduce from 375 mg:5 mL.

5. 325 mg:1 tablet

   Reduce from 975 mg:3 tablets.

6. a. 91.7%

   b. 125%

   c. 77.8%

7. a. 0.93

   Convert the fractional portion of the mixed number into the decimal 0.5. This now becomes 92.5%. Removing the percent sign and dividing by 100, the decimal equivalent is 0.925. Rounding to the hundredths place, the answer is finally expressed as 0.93.

   b. 0.13

   c. 1.05

8. a. 11:50

   22% is initially expressed as 22/100. This is reduced to 11/50, which is converted to the ratio of 11:50.

   b. 3:2

   150% may be expressed as 150/100. Dividing both the numerator and denominator by 150, it becomes 3/2. Converting this fraction to a ratio, it becomes 3:2.

   c. 1:200

   The initial fraction is 0.5/100. Making both the numerator and denominator whole numbers by multiplying each by 10, this fraction becomes 5/1000. Reducing this fraction to its

lowest terms, it becomes 1/200. Finally, this fraction is converted to the ratio of 1:200.

9. 10.8%

   $54/500 = 0.108$

   Converting this fraction to a percentage, it becomes 10.8%.

10. $250/0.45 = 555.56$

    As a check, multiply $555.56 \times 45\%$.

11. 86.9

    $1.1 \times 79 = 86.9$

12. 10.8

    $0.9\% = 0.009; 0.009 \times 1200 = 10.8$

13. 676.92

    $88/0.13 = 676.92$. As a check, multiply $676.92 \times 13\%$.

14. a. $x = 50$

    b. $x = 10.5$

    c. $x = 40$

    d. $x = 8.25$

15. a. 1.5 fl oz

    b. 4.5 fl oz

    c. 22.5 mL

    d. 43.5 mL

16. 12.5 mL

    $5 \text{ mL}/1 \text{ tsp} = x \text{ mL}/2.5 \text{ tsp}$

17. 0.71%

18. 2.8%

19. Yes. The computed standard of error is 3.33%.

20. 3.5 mL

    $20 \text{ mg}/1 \text{ mL} = 70 \text{ mg}/x \text{ mL}$

Chapter 3 Quiz

Version A

1. yes

   The form is correct for a physician, and the number verification is valid.

2. yes

   The form is correct for a physician, and the number verification is valid. Keep in mind that the DEA number for this physician may have been issued when she had a different last name than her current one.

3. no

   The first letter of a physician's DEA number will never be "W."

4. no

   While the letters are appropriate, the checksum digit is incorrect.

5. yes

   The form is correct for a physician, and the number verification is valid.

6. 40 capsules

   QID is the abbreviation for four times a day, and the duration of the treatment is 10 days.

7. 19 tablets

   1 tablet four times daily on the first day; 1 tablet three times daily on days two and three; 1 tablet twice daily on days four to six; and 1 tablet daily on days seven to nine

8. 140 mL

   20 mL/day $\times$ 7 days

9. 20 mg/mL

   2% is 2 g/100 mL. Converting 2 g to 2000 mg, the expression becomes 2000 mg/100 mL. This expression can be reduced to 20 mg/mL.

10. two full weeks

    5 mL/dose $\times$ 3 doses/day = 15 mL per day; 240 mL/(15 mL/day) = 16 days; 16 days accounts for two full weeks, but not three.

11. 22 full days

    90 capsules/(4 capsules/day) = 22.5 days

12. 60 days

    Every 12 hours' dosing means that two doses are taken per day, spaced 12 hours apart. Therefore, 120 tablets/ (2 tablets/day) = 60 days

13. 30 days

    90 capsules/ (3 capsules/day) = 30 days

14. microgram

15. three times daily

16. before meals

17. both ears

18. immediately

19. after meals

20. no known drug allergies

Chapter 3 Quiz

Version B

1. no

   The checksum digit should be 6.

   7 + 4 + 5 = 16; 2 $\times$ (1 + 6 +8) = 30; 16 + 30 = 3<u>6</u>

2. yes

   The form is correct, as is the checksum digit of 4.

3. yes

   The form is correct, as is the checksum digit of 2.

4. no

   The first letter for a physician's DEA number should either be A or B.

5. no

   There are too many digits in this DEA number.

6. 60 tablets

   LX is the Roman numeral for 60.

7. 280 mL

   5 mL/dose $\times$ 4 doses/day $\times$ 14 days = 280 mL

8. 36 tablets

   There can be as many as 2 tablets taken 6 times daily for 3 full days, which accounts for 36 tablets.

9. 20 days

40 tablets/(2 tablets/day) = 20 days.

10. Place 2 drops in both ears four times a day as needed for itching.

11. Take 1 tablet by mouth three times a day before meals.

12. Place 3 drops in the left eye every 4 hours while awake for 3 days.

13. Take 1 to 2 capsules by mouth, every 6 hours as needed for dizziness.

14 nothing by mouth

15. grain(s)

16. dispense as written

17. every 8 hours

18. as directed

19. discontinue

20. both eyes

Chapter 4 Quiz

Version A

1. 3200 mg = 3.200 g = 3.2 g

2. 2.5 mg = 2500. mcg = 2500 mcg

3. 650 mg/x mcg = 1 mg/1000 mcg; 650 × 1000 = 650,000/1 = 650,000; x = 650,000 mcg

4. 2.5 L/x mL = 1 L/1000 mL; 2.5 × 1000 = 2500; 2500/1 = 2500; x = 2500 mL

5. 425 mg × 1 g/1000 mg = 425/1000 = 0.425 g

6. 3250 mL × 1L/1000 mL = 3250/1000 = 3.25 L

7. 40 mg/1 mL = 120 mg/x mL; 1 × 120 = 120; 120/40 = 3; x = 3 mL

8. 40 mg/1 mL = 200 mg/x mL; 1 × 200 = 200; 200/40 = 5; x = 5 mL

9. 1 kg/2.2 lb = x kg/40 lb; 1 × 40 = 40; 40/2.2 = 18.18; x = 18.18 kg; 18.18 kg × 2 mg/kg = 36.4 mg of gentamicin

10. 40 mg/1 mL = 36.4 mg/x mL; 1 × 36.4 = 36.4; 36.4/40 = 0.91; x = 0.91 mL

11. 10 mg/1 mL = x mg/6 mL; 10 × 6 = 60; 60/1 = 60; x = 60 mg

12. 10 mg/1 mL = 20 mg/x mL; 1 × 20 = 20; 20/10 = 2; x = 2 mL

13. 10 mg/1 mL = 40 mg/x mL; 1 × 40 = 40; 40/10 = 4; x = 4 mL

14. tid = 3 doses/day; 40 mg/1 dose = x mg/3 doses; 40 × 3 = 120; 120/1 = 120; x = 120 mg

15. 30 mL/1 dose = 360 mL/x doses; 1 × 360 = 360; 360/30 = 12; x = 12 doses

16. [12 years/12 years + 12 years] × 250; 12/24 = 0.5; 0.5 × 250 = 125 mg

17. 80 lb/150 lb × 250; 80/150 = 0.533; 0.533 × 250 = 133.33 mg

18. 1 pt = 480 mL; 8 g = 8000 mg

8000 mg/480 mL = x mg/5 mL; 8000 × 5 = 40,000; 40,000/480 = 83.333; x = 83.333, rounded to 83.33 mg

19. 10 mg/2 mL = 8 mg/x mL; 2 × 8 = 16; 16/10 = 1.6; x = 1.6 mL

20. 10,000 units/1 mL = 25,000 units/x mL; 1 × 25,000 = 25,000; 25,000/10,000 = 2.5; x = 2.5 mL

Chapter 4 Quiz

Version B

1. 4800 mg = 4.800 g = 4.8 g

2. 5.2 mg = 5200. mcg = 5200 mcg

3. 325 mg/x mcg = 1 mg/1000 mcg; 325 × 1000 = 325,000; 325,000/1 = 325,000; x = 325,000 mcg

4. 4.5 mL/x mL = 1 L/1000 mL; 4.5 × 1000 = 4500; 4500/1 = 4500; x = 4500 mL

5. 155 mg × 1 g/1000 mg = 155/1000 = 0.155 g

6. 6250 mL × 1 L/1000 mL = 6250/1000 = 6.25 L

7. 40 mg/1 mL = 100 mg/x mL; 1 × 100 = 100; 100/40 = 2.5; x = 2.5 mL

8. 40 mg/1 mL = 250 mg/x mL; 1 × 250 = 250; 250/40 = 6.25; x = 6.25 mL

9. 1 kg/2.2 lb = x kg/60 lb; 1 × 60 = 60; 60/2.2 = 27.27; x = 27.27 kg; 27.27 kg × 3 mg/kg = 81.81 mg of gentamicin

10. 40 mg/1 mL = 81.81 mg/x mL; 1 × 81.81 = 81.81; 81.81/40 = 2.045; x = 2.045 mL, rounded to 2.05 mL

11. 10 mg/1 mL = x mg/5 mL; 10 × 5 = 50; 50/1 = 50; x = 50 mg

12. 10 mg/1 mL = 30 mg/x mL; 1 × 30 = 30; 30/10 = 3; x = 3 mL

13. 10 mg/1 mL = 20 mg/x mL; 1 × 20 = 20; 20/10 = 2; x = 2 mL

14. tid = 3 doses/day; 20 mg/1 dose = x mg/3 doses; 20 × 3 = 60; 60/1 = 60; x = 60 mg

15. 30 mL/1 dose = 480 mL/x doses; 1 × 480 = 480; 480/30 = 16; x = 16 doses

16. [6 years/6 years + 12 years] × 250; 6/18 = 0.333; 0.333 × 250 = 83.333, rounded to 83.33 mg

17. 40 lb/150 lb × 250; 40/150 = 0.266; 0.266 × 250 = 66.5 mg

18. 1 pt = 480 mL; 8 g = 8000 mg

8000 mg/480 mL = x mg/30 mL; 8000 × 30 = 240,000; 240,000/480 = 500; x = 500 mg

19. 10 mg/2 mL = 6 mg/x mL; 2 × 6 = 12; 12/10 = 1.2; x = 1.2 mL

20. 20,000 units/1 mL = 25,000 units/x mL; 1 × 25,000 = 25,000; 25,000/20,000 = 1.25; x = 1.25 mL

Chapter 5 Quiz

Version A

1. 1 pt = 480 mL; 1 tbsp = 15 mL

250 mg/15 mL = x mg/480 mL; 250 × 480 = 120,000; 120,000/15 = 8000; x = 8000 mg

2. 125 mg/5 mL = 500 mg/x mL; 5 × 500 = 2500; 2500/125 = 20; x = 20 mL

3. tid = 3 doses per day

500 mg/1 dose = x mg/3 doses; 500 × 3 = 1500; 1500/1 = 1500; x = 1500 mg

4. 1500 mg/1 day = x mg/10 days; 1500 × 10 = 15,000; 15,000/1 = 15,000; x = 15,000 mg

5. °F = (1.8 × 42) + 32; 1.8 × 42 = 75.6; 75.6 + 32 = 107.6 °F

6. °F = (1.8 × 70) + 32; 1.8 × 70 = 126; 126 + 32 = 158 °F

7. °C = (98.6 − 32)/1.8; 98.6 − 32 = 66.6; 66.6/1.8 = 37 °C

8. °C = (32 − 32)/1.8; 32 − 32 = 0; 0/1.8 = 0 °C

9. 80 mg/15 mL = 100 mg/x mL; 15 × 100 = 1500; 1500/80 = 18.75; x = 18.75 mL

10. q6h = 4 doses per day

100 mg/1 dose = x mg/4 doses; 100 × 4 = 400; 400/1 = 400; x = 400 mg

11. 1 kg/2.2 lb = x kg/150 lb; 1 × 150 = 150; 150/2.2 = 68.1818; x = 68.1818 kg, rounded to 68.18 kg

12. 1 kg/2.2 lb = x kg/75 lb; 1 × 75 = 75; 75/2.2 = 34.0909; x = 34.0909 kg, rounded to 34.09 kg

13. 1 kg/2.2 lb = x kg/200 lb; 1 × 200 = 200; 200/2.2 = 90.909; x = 90.909 kg, rounded to 90.91 kg

14. 1 kg/2.2 lb = 25 kg/x lb; 2.2 × 25 = 55; 55/1 = 55; x = 55 lb

15. 1 kg/2.2 lb = 38 kg/x lb; 2.2 × 38 = 83.6; 83.6/1 = 83.6; x = 83.6 lb

16. 1 kg/2.2 lb = 80 kg/x lb; 2.2 × 80 = 176; 176/1 = 176; x = 176 lb

17. 1 tsp = 5 mL

1 tsp/5 mL = 0.5 tsp/x mL; 5 × 0.5 = 2.5; 2.5/1 = 2.5; x = 2.5 mL

18. bid = 2 doses per day

2.5 mL/1 dose = x mL/2 doses; 2.5 × 2 = 5; 5/1 = 5; x = 5 mL

19. 5 mL/1 day = x mL/14 days; 5 × 14 = 70; 70/1 = 70; x = 70 mL

20. 10 mg/1 mL = x mg/70 mL; 10 × 70 = 700; 700/1 = 700; x = 700 mg

Chapter 5 Quiz

Version B

1. 1 cup = 240 mL

1 tbsp = 15 mL

250 mg/15 mL = x mg/240 mL; 250 × 240 = 60,000; 60,000/15 = 4000; x = 4000 mg

2. 125 mg/5 mL = 125 mg/x mL; 5 × 125 = 625; 625/125 = 5; x = 5 mL

   The label inserted is 125 mg/5 mL; therefore, 125 mg/5 mL = 125 mg/x mL; x = 5 mL

3. tid = 3 doses per day

   125 mg/1 dose = x mg/3 doses; 125 × 3 = 375; 375/1 = 375; x = 375 mg

4. 375 mg/1 day = x mg/10 days; 375 × 10 = 3750; 3750/1 = 3750; x = 3750 mg

5. °F = (1.8 × 54) + 32; 1.8 × 54 = 97.2; 97.2 + 32 = 129.2 °F

6. °F = (1.8 × 72) + 32; 1.8 × 72 = 129.6; 129.6 + 32 = 161.6 °F

7. °C = (100 − 32)/1.8; 100 − 32 = 68; 68/1.8 = 37.777, rounded to 37.78 °C

8. °C = (68 − 32)/1.8; 68 − 32 = 36; 36/1.8 = 20 °C

9. 1 tsp = 5 mL

   1 tsp/5 mL = 0.5 tsp/x mL; 5 × 0.5 = 2.5; 2.5/1 = 2.5; x = 2.5 mL

10. bid = 2 doses per day

    2.5 mL/1 dose = x mL/2 doses; 2.5 × 2 = 5; 5/1 = 5; x = 5 mL

11. 5 mL/1 day = x mL/14 days; 5 × 14 = 70; 70/1 = 70; x = 70 mL

12. 10 mg/1 mL = x mg/70 mL; 10 × 70 = 700; 700/1 = 700; x = 700 mg

13. 80 mg/15 mL = 100 mg/x mL; 15 × 100 = 1500; 1500/80 = 18.75; x = 18.75 mL

14. q6h = 4 doses per day

    100 mg/1 dose = x mg/4 doses; 100 × 4 = 400; 400/1 = 400; x = 400 mg

15. 1 kg/2.2 lb = x kg/155 lb; 1 × 155 = 155; 155/2.2 = 70.4545, rounded to 70.45 kg

16. 1 kg/2.2 lb = x kg/70 lb; 1 × 70 = 70; 70/2.2 = 31.8181, rounded to 31.82 kg

17. 1 kg/2.2 lb = x kg/210 lb; 1 × 210 = 210; 210/2.2 = 95.4545, rounded to 95.45 kg

18. 1 kg/2.2 lb = 20 kg/x lb; 2.2 × 20 = 44; 44/1 = 44; x = 44 lb

19. 1 kg/2.2 lb = 36 kg/x lb; 2.2 × 36 = 79.2; 79.2/1 = 79.2; x = 79.2 lb

20. 1 kg/2.2 lb = 81 kg/x lb; 2.2 × 81 = 178.2; 178.2/1 = 178.2; x = 178.2 lb

Chapter 6 Quiz

Version A

1. 50 mg/1 mL = 150 mg/x mL; 1 × 150 = 150; 150/50 = 3; x = 3 mL

2. 1 g = 1000 mg

   1000 mg/5 mL = 750 mg/x mL; 5 × 750 = 3750; 3750/1000 = 3.75; x = 3.75 mL

3. 10 mg/1 mL = x mg/50 mL; 10 × 50 = 500; 500/1 = 500; x = 500 mg

4. 1 g = 1000 mg

   1000 mg/10 mL = x mg/100 mL; 1000 × 100 = 100,000; 100,000/10 = 10,000; x = 10,000 mg

5. 10 mg/50 mL = x mg/1 mL; 10 × 1 = 10; 10/50 = 0.2; x = 0.2 mg/mL

6. 10 mg/1 dose = x mg/3 doses; 10 × 3 = 30; 30/1 = 30; x = 30 mg

7. 50 mL/1 dose = x mL/3 doses; 50 × 3 = 150; 150/1 = 150; x = 150 mL

8. 1 g/100 mL = x g/1000 mL; 1 × 1000 = 1000; 1000/100 = 10; x = 10 g

9. 1 g = 1000 mg

   1000 mg/5000 mL = 250 mg/x mL; 5000 × 250 = 1,250,000; 1,250,000/1000 = 1250; x = 1250 mL

10. 200 mg/20 mL = 40 mg/x mL; 20 × 40 = 800; 800/200 = 4; x = 4 mL

11. q8h = 3 doses in 24 hr

    4 mL/1 dose = x mL/3 doses; 4 × 3 = 12; 12/1 = 12; x = 12 mL

12. 40 mg/1 dose = x mg/3 doses; 40 × 3 = 120; 120/1 = 120; x = 120 mg

13. 50 mL/1 dose = x mL/3 doses; 50 × 3 = 150; 150/1 = 150; x = 150 mL

14. 40 mg/50 mL $= x$ mg/1 mL; $40 \times 1 = 40$; $40/50 = 0.8$; $x = 0.8$ mg/mL

15. 120 mg/1 day $= x$ mg/5 days; $120 \times 5 = 600$; $600/1 = 600$; $x = 600$ mg

16. 40 mEq/20 mL $= 20$ mEq/x mL; $20 \times 20 = 400$; $400/40 = 10$; $x = 10$ mL

17. 1 L = 1000 mL

    20 mEq/1000 mL $= x$ mEq/1 mL; $20 \times 1 = 20$; $20/1000 = 0.02$; $x = 0.02$ mEq/mL

18. 1 L = 1000 mL

    20 mEq/1000 mL $= x$ mEq/3000 mL; $20 \times 3000 = 60{,}000$; $60{,}000/1000 = 60$; $x = 60$ mEq

19. 10,000 units/1 mL $= 25{,}000$ units/x mL; $25{,}000 \times 1 = 25{,}000$; $25{,}000/10{,}000 = 2.5$; $x = 2.5$ mL

20. 10 units + 15 units = 25 units per day

    100 units/1 mL $= 25$ units/x mL; $1 \times 25 = 25$; $25/100 = 0.25$; $x = 0.25$ mL

Chapter 6 Quiz

Version B

1. 50 mg/1 mL $= 150$ mg/x mL; $1 \times 150 = 150$; $150/50 = 3$; $x = 3$ mL

2. 10 mg/50 mL $= x$ mg/1 mL; $10 \times 1 = 10$; $10/50 = 0.2$; $x = 0.2$ mg/mL

3. 10 mg/1 dose $= x$ mg/3 doses; $10 \times 3 = 30$; $30/1 = 30$; $x = 30$ mg

4. 50 mL/1 dose $= x$ mL/3 doses; $50 \times 3 = 150$; $150/1 = 150$; $x = 150$ mL

5. 1 g = 1000 mg

    1000 mg/10 mL $= 750$ mg/x mL; $10 \times 750 = 7500$; $7500/1000 = 7.5$; $x = 7.5$ mL

6. 100 mg/1 mL $= x$ mg/50 mL; $100 \times 50 = 5000$; $5000/1 = 5000$; $x = 5000$ mg

7. 1 g = 1000 mg

    1000 mg/10 mL $= x$ mg/250 mL; $1000 \times 250 = 250{,}000$; $250{,}000/10 = 25{,}000$; $x = 25{,}000$ mg

8. 1 g/100 mL $= x$ g/500 mL; $1 \times 500 = 500$; $500/100 = 5$; $x = 5$ g

9. 1 g = 1000 mg

    1000 mg/5000 mL $= 750$ mg/x mL; $5000 \times 750 = 3{,}750{,}000$; $3{,}750{,}000/1000 = 3750$; $x = 3750$ mL

10. 200 mg/20 mL $= 20$ mg/x mL; $20 \times 20 = 400$; $400/200 = 2$; $x = 2$ mL

11. q8h = 3 doses in 24 hr

    2 mL/1 dose $= x$ mL/3 doses; $2 \times 3 = 6$; $6/1 = 6$; $x = 6$ mL

12. 20 mg/1 dose $= x$ mg/3 doses; $20 \times 3 = 60$; $60/1 = 60$; $x = 60$ mg

13. 50 mL/1 dose $= x$ mL/3 doses; $50 \times 3 = 150$; $150/1 = 150$; $x = 150$ mL

14. 20 mg/50 mL $= x$ mg/1 mL; $20 \times 1 = 20$; $20/50 = 0.4$; $x = 0.4$ mg/mL

15. 60 mg/1 day $= x$ mg/5 days; $60 \times 5 = 300$; $300/1 = 300$; $x = 300$ mg

16. 40 mEq/20 mL $= 30$ mEq/x mL; $20 \times 30 = 600$; $600/40 = 15$; $x = 15$ mL

17. 1 L = 1000 mL

    30 mEq/1000 mL $= x$ mEq/1 mL; $30 \times 1 = 30$; $30/1000 = 0.03$; $x = 0.03$ mEq/mL

18. 1 L = 1000 mL

    30 mEq/1000 mL $= x$ mEq/3000 mL; $30 \times 3000 = 90{,}000$; $90{,}000/1000 = 90$; $x = 90$ mEq

19. 20,000 units/1 mL $= 25{,}000$ units/x mL; $25{,}000 \times 1 = 25{,}000$; $25{,}000/20{,}000 = 1.25$; $x = 1.25$ mL

20. 10 + 15 + 25 = 50 units per day

    100 units/1 mL $= 50$ units/x mL; $1 \times 50 = 50$; $50/100 = 0.5$; $x = 0.5$ mL

Chapter 7 Quiz

Version A

1. 5% = 5 g/100 mL

    5 g/100 mL $= x$ g/600 mL; $5 \times 600 = 3000$; $3000/100 = 300$; $x = 30$ g

2. NS = 0.9 g/100 mL

    0.9 g/100 mL $= x$ g/250 mL; $0.9 \times 250 = 225$; $225/100 = 2.25$; $x = 2.25$ g

3. $x\%/100$ mL $= 50$ g/500 mL; $100 \times 50 =$ 5000; 5000/500 $= 10$; $x\% = 10\%$

4. 100 mg $= 0.1$ g

   $x\%/100$ mL $= 0.1$ g/10 mL; $100 \times 0.1 = 10$; 10/10 $= 1$; $x\% = 1\%$

5. $7\% = 7$ g/100 mL; 7 g of dextrose/100 mL of fluid or 7 g/100 mL

6. 1 L $= 1000$ mL

   1000/75 $= 13.33$; 13.33 hr or approximately 13 hr and 20 min

7. 1000/100 $= 10$; 24/10 $= 2.4$, rounded up to 3; 3 bags

8. 1 L $= 1000$ mL

   1000/24 $= 41.666$, rounded to 41.7 mL/hr

9. 500 mg/4 hr $= x$ mg/1 hr; $500 \times 1 = 500$; 500/4 $= 125$; $x = 125$ mg/hr

10. 3 hr $= 180$ min

    500 mL/180 min $\times$ 15 gtts/mL; 500/180 $= 2.78$; $2.78 \times 15 = 41.7$, rounded down to 41 gtts/min

11. 40 mL/60 min $\times$ 20 gtts/mL; 40/60 $= 0.667$; $0.667 \times 20 = 13.33$, rounded down to 13; 13 gtts/min

12. 800 mg/250 mL $= 3.2$ mg/mL; 3.2 mg/mL $\div$ 15 gtts/mL $= 0.21$; 0.21 mg/gtt

13. D5 $= 5$ g/100 mL; 5 g/100 mL $= x$ g/1000 mL; $5 \times 1000 = 5000$; 5000/100 $= 50$; $x = 50$ g

14. 1000/125 $= 8$; 24/8 $= 3$; 50 g/1 bag $= x$ g/3 bags; $50 \times 3 = 150$; 150/1 $= 150$; $x = 150$ g

15. NS $= 0.9$ g/100 mL

    0.9 g/100 mL $= x$ g/ 1000 mL; $0.9 \times 1000 = 900$; 900/100 $= 9$; $x = 9$ g

16. 1000/125 $= 8$; 24/8 $= 3$; 9 g/1 bag $= x$ g/ 3 bags; $9 \times 3 = 27$; 27/1 $= 27$; $x = 27$ g

17. 40 mEq/1 bag $= x$ mEq/3 bags; $40 \times 3 = 120$; 120/1 $= 120$; $x = 120$ mEq

18. $D_5W = 5$ g/100 mL

    5 g/100 mL $= x$ g/10 mL; $5 \times 10 = 50$; 50/100 $= 0.5$; $0.5 \times 24 = 12$; 12 g

19. 1 g $= 1000$ mg

    1000 mg/250 mL $= x$ mg/10 mL; $1000 \times 10 = 10,000$; 10,000/250 $= 40$; $40 \times 24 = 960$; 960 mg

20. 10 mL/1 hr $= x$ mL/24 hr; $10 \times 24 = 240$; 240/1 $= 240$; $x = 240$ mL

Chapter 7 Quiz

Version B

1. NS $= 0.9$ g/100 mL

   0.9 g/100 mL $= x$ g/500 mL; $0.9 \times 500 = 450$; 450/100 $= 4.5$; $x = 4.5$ g

2. $D_{10}W = 10$ g/100 mL

   10 g/100 mL $= x$ g/700 mL; $10 \times 700 = 7000$; 7000/100 $= 70$; $x = 70$ g

3. 25 g/500 mL $= x$ g/ 100 mL; $25 \times 100 = 2500$; 2500/500 $= 5$; $x = 5$ g; 5 g/100 mL $= 5\%$

4. 9000 mg/60 mL $= x$ mg/100 mL; $9000 \times 100 = 900,000$; 900,000/60 $= 15,000$; 15,000/1000 $= 15$; 15%

5. 1000 mL $\div$ 100 mL/hr $= 10$ hr; 24 hr/10 hr $= 2.4$, rounded up to 3; 3 bags

6. $15\% = 15$ g/100 mL

   15 g of dextrose/100 mL of fluid or 15 g/100 mL

7. 1 L $= 1000$ mL

   1000 mL $\div$ 50 mL/hr $= 20$; 20 hr

8. 500 mg/4 hr $= x$ mg/1 hr; $500 \times 1 = 500$; 500/4 $= 125$ mg/hr

9. 500 mL/24 hr $= 20.833$, rounded to 20.83 mL/hr

10. 2 hr $= 120$ min

    250 mL/120 min $\times$ 15 gtts/mL; 250/120 $= 20.83$; $20.83 \times 15 = 31.35$, rounded down to 31 drops per minute; 31 gtts/min

11. 40 mL/60 min $\times$ 20 gtts/min; 40/60 $= 0.667$; $0.667 \times 20 = 13.33$, rounded down to 13 drops per minute; 13 gtts/min

12. 800 mg/250 mL $= 3.2$ mg/mL; 3.2 mg/mL $\div$ 15 gtts/mL $= 0.213$ mg/gtt

13. $D_5W = 5 \text{ g}/ 100 \text{ mL}$

5 g/ 100 mL = x g/10 mL; 5 × 10 = 50; 50/100 = 0.5; x = 0.5 g; 0.5 × 24 = 12; 12 g

14. 1 g = 1000 mg

1000 mg/250 mL = x mg/10 mL; 1000 × 10 = 10,000; 10,000/250 = 40; x = 40 mg; 40 × 24 = 960; 960 mg

15. 10 mL/1 hr = x mL/24 hr; 10 × 24 = 240; 240/1 = 240; x = 240 mL

16. $D_5 = 5 \text{ g}/100 \text{ mL}$

5 g/100 mL = x g/1000 mL; 5 × 1000 = 5000; 5000/100 = 50; x = 50 g

17. 1000/125 = 8; 24/8 = 3; 50 g/1 bag = x g/3 bags; 50 × 3 = 150; 150/1 = 150; x = 150 g

18. NS = 0.9 g/100 mL

0.9 g/100 mL = x g/1000 mL; 0.9 × 1000 = 900; 900/100 = 9; x = 9 g

19. 1000/125 = 8; 24/8 = 3; 9 g/1 bag = x g/ 3 bags; 9 × 3 = 27; 27/1 = 27; x = 27 g

20. 40 mEq/1 bag = x mEq/3 bags; 40 × 3 = 120; 120/1 = 120; x = 120 mEq

Chapter 8 Quiz

Version A

1. 3 + 62 = 65 parts total

3/65 = x/500; 3 × 500 = 1500; 1500/65 = 23.08; x = 23.08 mL of $D_{70}W$

70		3 parts of 70%
	8	
5		62 parts of 5%

2. 62/65 = x/500; 62 × 500 = 31,000; 31,000/65 = 476.92; x = 476.92 mL of D_5W

70		10 parts of 70%
	15	
5		55 parts of 5%

3. 10 parts

4. 55 parts

5. 65 parts

6. 10 + 55 = 65 total parts

10/65 = x/400; 10 × 400 = 4000; 4000/65 = 61.54; x = 61.54 mL of $D_{70}W$

7. 55/65 = x/400; 55 × 400 = 22,000; 22,000/65 = 338.46; x = 338.46 mL of D_5W

8. 3% = 3 g/100 g

3 g/100 g = x g/40 g; 3 × 40 = 120; 120/100 = 1.2; x = 1.2 g

9. 5 mg/1 mL = x mg/5 mL; 5 × 5 = 25; 25/1 = 25; x = 25 mg

10 mg/1 mL = 25 mg/x mL; 1 × 25 = 25; 25/10 = 2.5; x = 2.5 mL

5 − 2.5 = 2.5; 2.5 mL of gentamicin 10 mL stock solution; 2.5 mL of sterile water

10. 10 g/40 g × 100; 10/40 = 0.25; 0.25 × 100 = 25; 25%

11. 1500/70 × 15; 1500/70 = 21.43; 21.43 × 15 = 321.45; 321.45 mL

12. 1500/10 × 3; 1500 /10 = 150; 150 × 3 = 450; 450 mL

13. 1500/20 × 3; 1500/20 = 75; 75 × 3 = 225; 225 mL

14. 40 mEq/1 L = x mEq/1.5 L; 40 × 1.5 = 60; 4 mEq/1 mL = 60 mEq/x mL; 60/1 = 60; 60/4 = 15; 15 mL

15. 20 mEq/1 L = x mEq/1.5 L; 20 × 1.5 = 30; 3 mEq/1 mL= 30 mEq/x mL; 30/1 = 30; 30/3 = 10; 10 mL

16. 10 mM/1 L = x mM/1.5 L; 10 × 1.5 = 15; 3 mM/1 mL = 15 mM/x mL; 15/1 = 15; 15/3 = 5; 5 mL

17. 3 mM/1 L = x mM/1.5 L; 3 × 1.5 = 4.5; 3 mM/1 mL=4.5 mM/x mL; 4.5/1 = 4.5; 4.5/ 3 = 1.5; 1.5 mL

18. 10 mEq/1 L = x mEq/1.5 L; 10 × 1.5 = 15; 4.06 mEq/1 mL=15 mEq/x mL; 15/1 = 15; 15/4.06 = 3.69; 3.69 mL

19. MVI = 10 mL

20. $321.45 + 450 + 225 + 15 + 15 + 5 + 1.5 + 3.69 + 10 = 1046.64$; $1500 - 1046.64 = 453.36$; QSAD to 1500 mL with 453.36 mL of sterile water

Chapter 8 Quiz

Version B

1. $2.5 + 62.5 = 65$ parts total

   $2.5/65 = x/1000$; $2.5 \times 1000 = 2500$; $2500/65 = 38.46$; $x = 38.46$ mL of $D_{70}W$

2. $62.5/65 = x/1000$; $62.5 \times 1000 = 62{,}500$; $62{,}500/65 = 961.54$; $x = 961.54$ mL of D_5W

70		2.5 parts of 70%
	7.5	
5		62.5 parts of 5%

3. 13 parts

4. 52 parts

5. 65 parts

6. $13 + 52 = 65$ parts total

   $13/65 = x/700$; $13 \times 700 = 9100$; $9100/65 = 140$; $x = 140$ mL

7. $52/65 = x/700$; $52 \times 700 = 36{,}400$; $36{,}400/65 = 560$; $x = 560$ mL

70		13 parts of 70%
	18	
5		52 parts of 5%

8. $5\% = 5$ g/100 g

   5 g/100 g $= x$ g/50 g; $5 \times 50 = 250$; $250/100 = 2.5$; $x = 2.5$ g

9. 8 g/42 g $\times 100$; $8/42 = 0.19$; $0.19 \times 100 = 19$; 19%

10. 1 mg/1 mL $= x$ mg/ 4 mL; $1 \times 4 = 4$; $4/1 = 4$; $x = 4$ mg

    4 mg/1 mL $= 4$ mg/ x mL; $1 \times 4 = 4$; $4/4 = 1$ mL Decadron 4 mg/ mL stock solution; $4 - 1 = 3$; 3 mL of sterile water

11. $1500/70 \times 12$; $1500/70 = 21.43$; $21.43 \times 12 = 257.14$; 257.14 mL of dextrose

12. $1500/10 \times 5$; $1500/10 = 150$; $150 \times 5 = 750$; 750 mL of Aminosyn

13. $1500/20 \times 2$; $1500/20 = 75$; $75 \times 2 = 150$; 150 mL of Liposyn

14. 40 mEq/1 L $= x$ mEq/1.5 L; $40 \times 1.5 = 60$; $60/1 = 60$; $60/4 = 15$; 15 mL

15. 20 mEq/1 L $= x$ mEq/1.5 L; $20 \times 1.5 = 30$; $30/1 = 30$; $30/2 = 15$ mL

16. 10 mM/1 L $= x$ mM/1.5 L; $10 \times 1.5 = 15$; $15/1 = 15$; $15/3 = 5$; 5 mL

17. 3 mM/1 L $= x$ mM/1.5 L; $3 \times 1.5 = 4.5$; $4.5/1 = 4.5$; $4.5/3 = 1.5$; 1.5 mL

18. 10 mEq/1 L $= x$ mEq/1.5 L; $10 \times 1.5 = 15$; $15/1 = 15$; $15/4.06 = 3.69$; 3.69 mL

19. MVI $= 10$ mL

20. $257.14 + 750 + 150 + 15 + 15 + 5 + 1.5 + 3.69 + 10 = 1207.33$; $1500 - 1207.33 = 292.67$; QSAD to 1500 mL with 292.67 mL of sterile water

Chapter 9 Quiz

Version A

1. The pharmacy's income must be $1,172,920.00.

   $155,000.00 + $51,000.00 + $23,000.00 + $6,000.00 + $4,000.00 + $2,000.00 + $4,000.00 + $4,000.00 + $750,000.00 = $994,000.00; $994,000.00 \times 0.18 = $178,920.00; $994,000.00 + $178,920.00 = $1,172,920.00

2. The percentage profit is 29.1%.

   $1,401,489.00 - $994,000.00 = $407,489.00; $407,489.00/$1,401,489.00 = 0.291; $0.291 \times 100 = 29.1$

3. The percentage profit is 16.6%.

$1,191,692.00 − $994,000 = $197,692.00; $197,692.00/$1,191,692.00 = 0.166; 0.166 × 100 = 16.6

4. The markup rate is 87%.

$6.50/100 tablets = $0.065; $0.065 × 30 = $1.95; $14.80 − $1.95 = $12.85/14.80 = 0.868; 0.868 × 100 = 86.8, rounded to 87%

5. The markup rate is 26%.

$83.50/500 tablets = $0.167; $0.167 × 100 = $16.70; $22.50 − $16.70 = $5.80; 5.80/22.50 = 0.2577; 0.2577 × 100 = 25.77, rounded to 26%

6. The markup rate is 75%.

$4.36/100 tablets = $0.0436; $0.0436 × 30 = $1.31; $5.25 − $1.31 = $3.94; 3.94/5.25 = 0.7505; 0.7505 × 100 = 75.05, rounded to 75%

7. The discounted selling price is $2.86.

$4.76 × 0.40 = $1.90; $4.76 − $1.90 = $2.86

8. The discounted selling price is $3.89.

$5.19 × 0.25 = $1.30; $5.19 − $1.30 = $3.89

9. The selling price is $187.20.

$12.00 × 0.30 = $3.60; $12.00 + $3.60 = $15.60; $15.60 × 12 = $187.20

10. The total amount that the HMO reimbursed for capitation fees is $2750.00.

$275.00 × 10 = $2750.00

11. The pharmacy's drug cost is $729.87.

$89.63 + $126.54 + $420.45 + $117.50 + $46.75 = $729.87

12. The pharmacy made a profit.

13. The pharmacy made a profit of $1949.13.

$2750.00 − $800.87 = $1949.13

14. The pharmacy's turnover rate is 3.32.

$585,000.00/$176,000.00 = 3.32

15. The annual depreciation is $900.00.

$5,000.00 − $500.00 = $4,500.00; $4,500.00/5 = $900.00

16. The pharmacy will submit $10.07 for reimbursement.

$82.00 × .03 = $2.46; $82.00 + $2.46 = $84.46; $84.46 /100 = 0.8446; 0.8446 × 6 = 5.068; $5.068 + $5.00 = $10.068, rounded to $10.07

Drug	Count/ Package Size	Minimum Par Level	Maximum Par Level	Current Inventory	Reorder Amount
17. cefaclor 500 mg tab	100	250	500	140	Three bottles of 100 tablets 500 − 140 = 360; 360/100 = 3.6
18. cefprozil 500 mg tab	50	30	100	34	None The inventory is greater than the minimum par level.
19. doxycycline 50 mg cap	50	30	200	100	None The inventory is greater than the minimum par level.
20. furosemide 40 mg tab	100	250	1000	107	Eight bottles of 100 tablets 1000 − 107 = 893; 893/100 = 8.93

Chapter 9 Quiz

Version B

1. The pharmacy's income must be $1,870,300.00.

   $278,000.00 + $122,000.00 + $50,000.00 + $6,000.00 + $4,000.00 + $2,000.00 + $4,000.00 + $4,000.00 + $1,115,000.00 = $1,585,000.00; $1,585,000.00 × 0.18 = $285,300.00; $1,585,000.00 + $285,300.00 = $1,870,300.00

2. The percentage profit is 51.5%.

   $2,401,489.00 − $1,585,000.00 = $816,489.00; $816,489.00/1,585,000.00 = 0.515; 0.515 × 100 = 51.5

3. The percentage profit is 25.7%.

   $1,991,692.00 − $1,585,000.00 = $406,692.00; $406,692.00/1,585,000.00 = 0.257; 0.257 × 100 = 25.7

4. The discounted selling price is $2.86.

   $4.76 × 0.40 = $1.90; $4.76 − $1.90 = $2.86

5. The discounted selling price is $3.89.

   $5.19 × 0.25 = $1.30; $5.19 − $1.30 = $3.89

6. The selling price is $187.20.

   $12.00 × 0.30 = $3.60; $12.00 + $3.60 = $15.60; $15.60 × 12 = $187.20

7. The markup rate is 87%.

   $6.50/100 tablets = $0.065; $0.065 × 30 = $1.95; $14.80 − $1.95 = 12.85/14.80 = 0.868; 0.868 × 100 = 86.8, rounded to 87%

8. The markup rate is 26%.

   $83.50/500 tablets = $0.167; $0.167 × 100 = $16.70; $22.50 − $16.70 = $5.80; 5.80/22.50 = 0.2577;

   0.2577 × 100 = 25.77, rounded to 26%

9. The markup rate is 75%.

   $4.36/100 tablets = $0.0436; $0.0436 × 30 = $1.31; $5.25 − $1.31 = $3.94; 3.94/5.25 = 0.750; 0.750 × 100 = 75%

10. The total amount that the HMO reimbursed for capitation fees is $2325.00.

    $155.00 × 15 = $2325.00

11. The pharmacy's drug cost is $862.97.

    $89.63 + $126.54 + $420.45 + $117.50 + $46.75 + $27.23 + $34.87 = $862.97

12. The pharmacy made a profit.

13. The pharmacy made a profit of $1462.03.

    $2325.00 − $862.97 = $1462.03

14. The pharmacy's turnover rate is 3.18.

    $725,000.00/$228,050.00 = 3.179, rounded to 3.18

15. The annual depreciation is $1,400.00.

    $15,000.00 − $1000.00 = $14,000.00; $14,000.00/10 = $1,400.00

16. The pharmacy will submit $17.98 for reimbursement.

    $42.00 × .03 = $1.26; 42.00 + 1.26 = $43.26; $43.26 /100 = 0.4326: 0.4326 × 30 = 12.978: 12.98 + $5.00 = $17.98

Drug	Count/ Package Size	Minimum Par Level	Maximum Par Level	Current Inventory	Reorder Amount
17. metformin 500 mg tab	100	250	500	200	Three bottles of 100 tablets 500 − 200 = 300
18. citalopram 40 mg cap	100	150	300	130	One bottle of 100 tablets 300 − 130 = 170
19. raloxifene 60 mg cap	50	30	200	100	None Current inventory is greater than the minimum par level.
20. lisinopril 5 mg tab	100	250	500	260	None Current inventory is greater than the minimum par level.